THE

LEUKAEMIA DIARIES

Seeing the Funnier Side of Cancer

A. D. HYDE

ISBN: 9798594458383

Because of the dynamic nature of the Internet, any web addresses or links contained in this book may have changed since publication and may no longer be valid. The views expressed in this work are solely those of the author and do not necessarily reflect the views of the publisher, and the publisher hereby disclaims any responsibility for them.

The author of this book does not dispense medical advice or prescribe the use of any technique as a form of treatment for physical, emotional, or medical problems without the advice of a physician, either directly or indirectly. The intent of the author is only to offer information of a general nature to help you in your quest for emotional and spiritual well-being. In the event you use any of the information in this book for yourself, which is your constitutional right, the author and the publisher assume no responsibility for your actions.

Certain stock imagery © Getty Images.

British Cataloguing Publication Data: A catalogue record of this book is available from The British Library.

Also available on Kindle.

CONTENTS

INTRODUCTION

I have Lukemia? Or is it Leukemia....no...I think it's Leukaemia... bugger it...I have cancer of the blood, and this is a documentary of my journey from just before being diagnosed with Chronic Myeloid Leukaemia (CML), through the scary 'I'm going to die' bit, the joys of having bone marrow samples taken, chemotherapy, and then getting back to work and beyond.

I started writing this book because my wife said: "You really should write all this stuff down, it could help someone going through the same thing you are." I guess what she meant by 'all this stuff', was all the experiences and emotions I was going through and the way I was coping with them. Initially, I thought it would be a bit egotistical of me to write a book on cancer. After all, what could I possibly have to say that would be worth listening to, never mind worth buying a book for? But as time passed, I found myself talking to more and more people who were either suffering from some form of cancer or who had someone close to them who was affected. I began to realise that my outlook on cancer was different and my way of dealing with it was equally as unique, so perhaps I did have something useful to say.

With the realisation that I had cancer, came the debilitating devastation that left me feeling so cold, scared and alone. I could have easily curled up into a ball and just given up, but I didn't. Instead of letting the enormous task ahead overwhelm me, I did what I always do...I took baby steps and tackled my condition one step at a time. This gave me the strength to face each stage of my treatment with a smile on my face. Even in the darkest of times, I would always find something to laugh about (well, almost always). It wasn't bravado or some attempt to look cool and it certainly wasn't me ignoring the gravity of my situation. It was more instinctive. Over the years, I have trained myself not to waste time worrying. I see no point in the emotion; it serves no purpose and only succeeds in causing pain and anguish. The way I see it is, if something bad is on the horizon, you do all you can to prepare for it, then forget about it. If you've done all you can to prepare for it, will thinking about it every second of the day help? No, of course not. So why worry? Sounds simple I know, but with a little practice, it becomes second nature. That's why I found I could cope with my leukaemia so well. I knew that the doctors were doing their best to help me, so all I had to do was take the medication and follow a few lifestyle instructions. Would worrying about what might happen help my situation? No.

If your life has been touched by cancer, whether it's your own or a loved one's, you'll soon discover that you're not the only one. Whether it's a close friend or a colleague from work, you'll find most people will have a story to tell. There will be some sad stories, some inspirational stories and even some angry ones...all will be emotional, but even here you'll find humour. One of my favourite examples of this involved a friend who said, "I worked with two guys who had Leukaemia..." There was a pause after which, he said, quite matter of factly, "Of course they're both dead now." I looked at him just long enough for him to realise what he'd said, long enough for the horror to fill his face and Just as he a started to stutter his apology. I let him off the hook by bursting out with laugher, because let's face it... it was funny!

Although I talk about seeing the funny side, I must stress that being told you have cancer is probably the most frightening time of your life, it certainly was for me. Whether it happens to you or a loved one, I can assure you of one thing...you will handle it in your own unique way. You will go through a kaleidoscope of emotions ranging from horror, disbelief, fear, anger, helplessness, guilt, and many other dwarf names. You mustn't get consumed by these emotions. You need to come to terms with the shitty stick you have been handed. I had my breakdown, where I went through the first stage of disbelief, thinking it was a nightmare and that any second now I would wake up and life would be good again. I went through the stage of being terrified and feeling so alone and without hope. I went through the stage where I felt racked with guilt that I would be leaving my beautiful wife and daughters to fend for themselves. Finally, I confronted and came to terms with the possibility that I might die. All this happened in the space of 24 hours ... 24 head-spinning hours, after which I got up and said to myself, "F**k it!" There was no point in feeling sorry for myself because that wasn't going to do me or the people I love any good. I have always tried to see the funny side of life, so I thought...why change now? I went one step further, in that I also decided that I didn't want people to feel sorry for me. I didn't want people to say, "it's such a shame" or "I feel so sorry for him and his family." No, I wanted them to be inspired by me. I wanted them to say "wow, he is amazing".

In the early stages of writing this book, I gave the first few chapters to my wife to proofread (she's good at that sort of thing). She went off to another room to read it in private and after about 30 minutes I started to wonder if what I had written was so bad that she didn't want to tell me. It turned out that reading those chapters had brought back so many memories that she ended up sobbing into a pile of tissues. When she finally came back we just hugged each other and cried.

After composing ourselves, we started to discuss what I had written. We talked openly about the feelings that I couldn't possibly have told her at the time, which was exactly what I wanted from this book. She then paused for a few seconds and went on to say, "you talk about coming to terms with death as being the most important thing that you believe cancer sufferers should do, but you don't say how." I knew that the answer would upset her, but she was right, I had to put it down in words. I said to her that I knew I had some form of cancer many months before I told her. I explained that I was convinced I would die, but had pushed it to the back of my mind so we could have a wonderful 'last' Christmas together (she still tells me off for not going to the doctors straight away).

I went on to say that after eventually going to the doctor, I remembered kneeling in our bedroom while she was downstairs and I started to cry. I whispered over and over again "I am so sorry...so sorry...please forgive me "I wasn't talking to God, I was talking to her and our daughters. I was pleading in the darkness for their forgiveness for leaving them. I felt so much guilt it hurt. I then started to plead to any power that would listen "please don't let me die...please, I'll do anything, just let me stay with my family...please...please." I just kept repeating it over and over again. I was still whispering because I didn't want her to hear, I didn't want to burden her with such desperate emotions. After a while, my mind went blank and out of that blank darkness a question came to me "If you died tomorrow, would you have any regrets?" To which, I immediately replied... "yes, of course I would!" I never got to be an astronaut, I never learned how to move objects with the power of my mind, I never managed to complete that bloody Rubik's Cube, I never went on an expedition to the North Pole and there were more, lots more. But before I got too carried away, another thought came in to my mind: "think about all the wonderful memories you have and all the love you have in your life." So, I started to think of all the wonderful things I had done, the memories I had shared with my loved ones...with my wife, and then I thought back to that first question again..." If you died tomorrow, would you have any regrets?" This time my answer was different, it was a resounding no! I have had some truly wonderful times with wonderful people...so..." No, I have no regrets." As soon as I had said it out loud, the fear, the guilt and the heartache melted away to be replaced with a feeling of tranquillity. Now, that didn't mean that every time I thought about leaving my wife and daughters I was fine because I wasn't. What I am saying, is that I didn't let these emotions eat away at me inside. Dying wasn't something I wanted, but it was something I accepted. I don't expect everyone to come to this point as quickly or in the same manner as I did, but I hope this book will show you that it is possible and that it benefits not just you but your loved ones too.

My wife then said, "People are also going to ask where you got your strength and resilience from, so perhaps you should try and say something about that too?" ...well... I can remember the exact point where I discovered my inner strength and where I decided to develop a new outlook on life. Up until this particular point I believed that I had bad luck. I believed that I had to work so much harder than everyone else to get what I wanted in life. I believed that if I told anyone what I wanted or was hoping for, then fate would make sure that it was taken from me.

The incident involved a car I owned and loved. This was the car that I drove to my wedding day; this was the car that had safely transported both my children home from hospital after their births. It was so reliable...until it started not to be reliable. It was little things at first, then bigger and bigger things. It would break down regularly and each time the problem would be something different and increasingly more expensive. It got to the point that when I phoned the breakdown services they recognised me and said that I had broken down more than any of their other customers that year. Each time we had the car fixed, we thought that we could relax, but within weeks something else would go wrong. We couldn't afford a new car and we couldn't really afford the repair bills. Fortunately my father in law was a car mechanic and he did most of the repair work for free, and we just had to pay for the parts. The incident that changed my life was when I had been down to his garage to get yet another thing fixed on the car and I had just set off for home with my eldest daughter who was about 2 years old at the time. It was late at night and I was in the middle of nowhere when the car broke down again. I managed to get to a phone and contact Reg who came out to pick us up and took us back to his house. When we were safely back at the house and my daughter was being looked after by her grandmother, I remember looking out of the window and crying...I was broken, helpless and I didn't know what to do...I felt I was being punished and that now my children were suffering too. Then Reg came up with the bad news "I'm afraid it's going to need a new engine and it's going to be very expensive." That's when I realised something about myself, something that has given me strength ever since...and it's that I can be beaten. I will give up and concede defeat under overwhelming odds just like any normal person would. But on that night I discovered that unlike most people I respond differently if you kick me when I'm down. Seconds after Reg had given me the bad news about the car I thought 'No...that's enough...that's quite enough, I'd had about as much as I could take and I wasn't going to take anymore.' That was the last time I ever felt helpless. I stood up and started to discuss my options calmly with Reg, but was immediately interrupted by my daughter who had come over for a cuddle and to play the 'how far can I stick my finger up Daddies nose' game. I looked at her and thought 'how could I ever have believed that all I had was bad luck?'

From that point on I stopped believing in good or bad luck. I also stopped complaining about the weather, which is a national pastime in the UK. I started to appreciate everything in my life. Instead of complaining that the summer wasn't that hot, I started to appreciate that we had 4 wonderfully different seasons that each bring with them something new to celebrate and enjoy. My particular favourite is autumn, with its wonderful colours, Halloween, bonfire night, my birthday and the thought that Christmas is not that far away. I found myself enjoying gardening in the rain. I learnt that no matter how bad things get, there is always hope, you just have to look for it.

It's my sincere hope that in sharing my innermost thoughts and memories in this book that I can help people get through a terrible time in their lives.

Words of Wisdom: The biggest and most helpful words of wisdom I can share with you, is to face and come to terms with the possibility that you might die. Once you have done this, you'll find that your whole outlook changes and you can cope with just about anything.

CHAPTER 1

The beginning of something

It all started in the summer of 2016. I woke up one morning, went to the toilet as usual, but then proceeded to piss razor blades! "Oh bother" I said, or words to that effect. I didn't want to go to the doctors because I had gone there a few months previous with a similar issue, and they'd sent me to the hospital for a barrage of tests, which was just about the most humiliating and painful experience of my life. I remember leaving the hospital in such an emotional state that I cried. After all those tests, they concluded that they couldn't find anything wrong, other than the fact that I had a urine infection.

So, I vowed never to go through that again, which is why this time I decided not to go to the doctors. Instead, I went to everyone's trusty friend: 'the internet' or as we say in the north of England... T'internet. He would tell me what to do. He's never let me down...well...apart from that time he said I had pneumonia and it turned out to be a chest infection and then there was that time I was having a heart attack...and it turned out to be...another chest infection. You can't really blame him for my inability to input the correct set of symptoms, can you?

So, I opened my laptop and typed 'how to treat a urine infection' and his first reply was "if you are male and you suspect you have a urine infection, you should seek medical advice" ...He was quite adamant about it. I tried different words with different combinations. But each time he said: "if you're male, you *should really seek medical advice*" Well, we can skip that bit I thought...what does he say next? Well...er...not a lot if you are male. He just kept going on about how difficult it is for men to get urine infections and that it is often an indicator of something more serious...well, it can't be that difficult to get a urine infection because this was my second episode in twelve months!

Don't look like that...we can all be idiots and bury our heads in the sand when it comes to the blindingly obvious...And believe me, there is more of this type of thinking to come. Let's get back to DIY cures for my urine infection. He doesn't have much advice for men, but he's got loads for women. So let's follow the advice for women...what's the worst that could happen?

My friend T'internet said: "Drinking cider vinegar will kill the bacteria that cause urine infections." He showed me a quote by Susan from Texas who said: "Every time I get a urine infection, I drink cider vinegar in the morning and the evening, and after just a couple of days the infection is much better." Great I thought, I have some cider vinegar in the cupboard from that time I started to get acid reflux and the internet recommended I should drink vinegar last thing at night....it didn't work for that, but perhaps it would for this. After two days of smelling like a jar of pickled onions, the infection wasn't getting any better. My wife Debbie said, "You must see the doctor!" I reluctantly agreed and walked down to my local surgery and spoke to a rather scary old lady at the reception desk. "Could I see a doctor?" I said politely. "Oh, we're very busy, is it an emergency?" she said, looking at me as though I was a child. To which I replied that I suspected that it would be soon if I didn't see a doctor. I got a disapproving look, after which she asked, "What is the problem?" in front of a packed waiting room. I wanted to say, "Call me old fashioned, but I'd like to tell that to a qualified doctor in the privacy of their examination room and not to a receptionist in front of twelve complete strangers" What I actually said was "I'd rather tell the doctor if you don't mind." Well, that didn't go down well either. She looked at her computer and muttered something under her breath, then looked at her note pad, then back to the computer and finally said that she could fit me in next week. I then said that there was no way I could wait a week. "Well I suppose we could put you on the list for the emergency surgery this afternoon," she said in a rather annoyed voice. I said thank you and went into the waiting room. After an hour or so I finally got in to see the doctor. I explained my symptoms and he confirmed that I had a urine infection, but instead of going straight for the antibiotics prescription as I had hoped, he continued reading my notes on the computer screen. "You had a urine infection about 6 months ago, didn't you?" he said..." We should really send you for some tests at the hospital," he said. I immediately said that I did not want to repeat that experience and gave him the look (it always works on the kids.... well...sometimes). He reluctantly said "OK, let's put you on a course of antibiotics, but if you get another urine infection in the next twelve months we must investigate further because it could be an indicator of something more serious. What could he be thinking about? Possibly the fact that if you have a weakened immune system you are more susceptible to getting urine infections...and having something like Leukaemia will weaken your immune system...interesting...it all seems so obvious now.

The next day Debbie and I were off to a wedding in Lille, France. Originally Debbie was concerned that I wouldn't be

3

able to come because I was ill, but armed with my freshly prescribed antibiotics I said I would be OK...what's the worst that could happen? Well, where do I start? It didn't help that Lille was in the grips of a mini heat wave with temperatures in excess of forty degrees Celsius. The heat would have been uncomfortable if I was fit and healthy, but with my 'infection' it was unbearable. At least I thought it was just because of my infection, one of the side effects of having Leukaemia is excessive sweating, especially at night. Wherever we went I would first have to find the nearest air conditioning unit or window and sit as close as possible to it, otherwise, I would just drip with sweat and feel so sick. The first day was really bad, but as the wedding was on the following day, I hoped that the antibiotics would start doing their job and I would be able to enjoy the day. Unfortunately, when I awoke on the day of the wedding, I felt worse and when I say I felt worse...I mean much worse. I managed to make it through the wedding ceremony...just. All I needed to do was get through the dinner and then I could get some rest before the evening celebrations, or so I thought. This wedding was different. This wedding was packed with organised events from the ceremony right through till the early hours of the following morning. A day of organised celebrations would have been amazing if I wasn't so unwell. But I was very unwell and there was no chance to sneak away for a rest. It was one of the longest most torturous days I think I have ever experienced, closely followed by an equally tortuous evening.

Skip to the next day and we arrive back at home in the UK to see that there was a message on the house phone. It was a message from the doctor. "Hello, Mr Hyde? ...We have the results of your urine test and unfortunately the antibiotics I prescribed for you will not work against the infection you have.

Could you please come back to the surgery as soon as possible to pick up a new prescription?" The message was three days old and it was a Sunday, and the next day was a bank holiday. So I had to wait another two days before I could start a new course of antibiotics. I managed to get through those two days and after another week of antibiotics, the infection was finally gone. I had lost six kilograms in weight over this period, which was a good thing. But instead of feeling good about life, I felt...well...not quite right.

I started back at the gym and playing squash, but I just didn't seem to have as much energy as before. I put this down to being on antibiotics for an extended period. My muscles and joints ached pretty much all the time, and I started bruising very easily. All I had to do was bump gently into a door handle and a huge purple bruise would appear in a matter of minutes. Another couple of symptoms of Leukaemia, the first is fatigue/tiredness and the second is bruising easily...If I were a medical professional, I would be getting suspicious by now.

A month later and I still felt the same. I kept saying to Debbie that I didn't feel right, she would encourage me to see the doctor. Of course, I took this advice and put it on my 'must-do' list, then went to my old friend the Internet or as he likes to be called T'internet. I put all my symptoms into one of those medical diagnosis programs and he said that I had either "Stomach cancer...A brain tumour...Underactive thyroid gland or A vitamin deficiency"...of course! ...it was obvious... I had a vitamin deficiency! So, I started taking various combinations of vitamins and it wasn't long before...yes you guessed it...nothing changed.

It was November 2016 when I was lying in bed and admiring my flat and firm stomach (I had lost eighteen kilograms by this point. I remember thinking that all the hard work down the gym was paying off and under the fat, I was developing a six-pack! Unfortunately, I noticed something strange about my firm stomach. It wasn't so much a '6 pack', but more like a '3 pack.' The left-hand side of my stomach was indeed rock hard, but the right-hand side was...well...flabby. Another symptom of leukaemia is an enlarged spleen, which causes stomach discomfort, bloatedness and in extreme cases...a firm abdomen...if I was a medical professional, I would be really suspicious by now. Something was really wrong! I should, of course, have arranged to see the doctor straight away, which is why I immediately went to my old friend T'internet. So, I pulled out my smartphone and put in my symptoms and he said: "A rigid abdomen is often the sign of an underlying condition such as stomach cancer." In actual fact, most of the articles said the same thing. I looked up the survival rates for stomach cancer and it wasn't pleasant reading. So, I thought a little bit of reverse psychology is required here...I thought if I convinced myself that I did indeed have cancer, then when I went to the doctors he would tell me I was stupid and that in actual fact I had a simple case of cramp or something equally benign. The trouble was...that deep down...I knew I had cancer.

Christmas is a big thing to me and my family (mostly to me). Every year I take 2-3 weeks off work and I make sure we have the best Christmas ever. I didn't and don't want my children to associate Christmas with me having cancer and dying. I want them to always associate Christmas with twinkly lights, decorations, great food, fun, family and love. So, I decided that if this was to be my last Christmas, it would be the best ever (I told you there were more amazing decisions to come, didn't I?). I decided that I would go to the doctors in January. I can hear you shouting "are you stupid?! You can't wait! See the doctor now!" Here's the thing, even now I ask myself the question 'Would I do the same thing if I could go back in time knowing what I know now?' and unbelievably I hear myself saying 'yes'.

We had the best Christmas ever, full of family, friends, fun and love. I was still losing weight so I felt really good about my body. Like many men, I had let the weight pile on over my 30s and 40s and was continually trying to lose weight. After losing over six kilograms during the time I was on antibiotics I decided to make a supreme effort to keep it off, so I cut down the size of my meals, no seconds and no eating after 7 pm. The real reason for not eating after 7 pm was because in the last 6 months I started to have real problems with acid reflux. It would generally occur in the middle of the night when I would wake up not being able to breathe. Some food/liquid would come up my airway and then into my windpipe, which would close as a defence mechanism. I would dash out of bed screeching loudly as I tried, unsuccessfully, to breathe. I would run into the bathroom and attempt to clear my windpipe by coughing. This was extremely difficult because I would have hardly any air in my lungs. It would usually take anything from thirty seconds to a heart-stopping sixty seconds to get to the point where I could breathe again. I remember going to see a doctor when it started and all he had to say was that I should lose weight.

Looking back now I can see that the acid reflux, fatigue, aching muscles and bruising were all connected to my Leukaemia. Even after the excesses of Christmas, I was still losing weight. I was now nearly twenty-four kilograms lighter and had dropped nine centimetres off my waist. It was twenty years since I'd been this weight, but I couldn't really enjoy it because I felt so fatigued. I'm good at putting things to one side and not thinking about them. So the cancer issue did not affect my enjoyment over Christmas. But every now and again I would look over at Debbie (who was my first and only love) and wonder whether this would be the last Christmas I would spend with her. Then I would look at my daughters...well...all I could think about was who would be there to protect them after I was gone? When they were very young, I told them that I would always protect them. I told them that I had a magical power that meant I could put an invisible bubble around them to protect them, even when I wasn't with them. So, this Christmas, I made them each a present to remind them of their protective bubble. I wanted them to feel as though I was there ...after... well after I was gone. Christmas went the way I wanted it to, but the festivities inevitably ended. Then came January and the start of a New Year and potentially my last year. So as I promised, I arranged an appointment with the doctor.

Words of Wisdom (WoW): If you think something is wrong with you...do not open your laptop...see the doctor and don't put it off. I was lucky, but my CML could have progressed to a stage that was not easily treated and I could easily have died. I also could have ruptured my spleen...and died.

Chapter 2

The doctors

The day of the appointment came, I told Debbie that I was just having a check-up. I didn't want her to worry unnecessarily. I must admit I was in a bit of a daze that day, so much so, that I couldn't even remember how I got there. I just remember sitting in the crowded doctor's waiting room. Doctor's waiting rooms can be depressing places. After all, you don't go there because you're fit and healthy, do you? That afternoon the place was already packed when I arrived. I always like to people watch when I'm waiting, and try to guess what ailments they have. There was an old woman near the door who kept moaning in agony, but instead of feeling sorry for her, I just thought if you're that ill why don't you go to the hospital? There was an old man in the corner bent over with his hands on his knees and breathing with great difficulty. Every now and then he looked up with a desperate and pained look in his eyes. There were the compulsory teenagers glued to their smartphones with accompanying adults trying unsuccessfully to hold a conversation with them. Then there was the first-time mother and her young child, with her holistic approach to parenting. This is the type of parent who would hold a calm conversation with their child, even if the child was stabbing their pet hamster: "Now Rupert, do we think that it's a good or bad thing to be stabbing one's pet hamster?" This particular toddler was called Jocasta and she would walk up to people in the waiting room one by one and would turn to her mum to ask an annoying or inappropriate question. For example:

- "Mummy, mummy, mummy why does that man have his hand wrapped up in a towel?" she asked. "Well darling, he's hurt his hand and is in a lot of pain, but the doctor is going to make it all better" her mum would reply.
- "Mummy, mummy, mummy...why is that man making noises?" she asked. "He's got asthma, do you remember your cousin Isabel? She has asthma" her mum would reply.
- "Mummy, mummy, mummy...why is that man so fat?" she asked. "Darling, we don't say fat, that's not polite, we say overweight" her mother said while smiling at the man.

All the time this was going on, I was waiting for the little girl to turn her attention to me and ask "Mummy, mummy, mummy what's wrong with him?" ...to which I would have shouted "I have cancer and I'm going to die!" But before she could get to me, my name was called out and I made my way to the doctor's room.

It was at this point that reality came flooding in, this is real now. I am officially acknowledging that there is something wrong with me and that it is most probably cancer. I walked into the doctor's room, where a smartly dressed elderly gentleman was awaiting my arrival. He was wearing a tweed suit with a matching waistcoat. He had a professional manner, which is another way of saying that he wasn't good with people. I explained why I was there and he asked me a few questions. He raised an eyebrow as I told him when I first noticed something was wrong. He didn't say anything, but I'm sure he was wondering why I had left it this late before coming in. He then asked me to jump up on the examination table and proceeded to examine me. It wasn't long before his professional cold exterior changed as he started to look concerned. "I think we need to take a blood sample and send it off to the hospital...tonight" he paused. Then he said, "I'll be frank with you Mr Hyde, it looks like you have an enlarged spleen and this is most likely going to be an indication of something much more serious." He then gave me a bloods form and asked me to take it to the receptionist and said that I should say that I need to have the bloods taken now. Off I went to reception, where I passed on the message to the receptionist. "Oh," she said in an annoyed voice "The nurse isn't in today, you'll have to come in tomorrow." I said that the doctor was insistent that the bloods should be taken tonight. She 'tutted' and picked up the phone to talk to the doctor. When he answered, she told him what she had told me and before she had put the phone down the doctor was there by my side. "OK Mr Hyde, come with me and I'll take the blood sample." He then looked over at the receptionist and said: "Once I have taken Mr Hyde's bloods, could you see that they are sent off to the hospital straight away." The receptionist nodded and her face changed immediately, going from superior smugness to genuine concern.

The next thing I remember is walking through the front door of my home. I had decided not to tell Debbie, after all, why put her through any unnecessary pain? I planned to walk into the kitchen and say everything was OK. So, I did exactly that, I walked into the kitchen where she was working. She looked up from her computer and asked me casually if everything was OK? And just as I planned...I broke down in tears and blubbered out that I was scared. Well, that went well I thought. I explained the whole story and rather than her being angry that I had kept it from her, she was brilliant. She saw the fear in my face and was positive and strong. Even though I'm sure inside, her world was caving in. After crying in her arms for a while I felt much better. I think I felt better partly because of the hug and partly for finally sharing the secret with her. After regaining my composure, I said, "Well, there's nothing I can do about it, I'm off to play squash" (which on retrospect with an enlarged spleen was not the wisest thing to have done). After winning a rather exhausting game with a colleague from work, I felt calm and refreshed. This game would also give me some ammunition to tease him in the months to come. I could not only say that he was beaten by someone twice his age, but also by someone with an enlarged spleen and in the advanced stages of Leukaemia.

When I got home, I settled down with Debbie in front of the TV with a cup of tea and started to watch a movie. Within minutes of sitting down the house phone rang. This was unusual, because we rarely got calls on the house phone. The only calls we got were scams from people who said they were from Microsoft saying that our computer has messaged Microsoft directly to say that it has been infected by a software virus and that for a fee they will fix it for me (how kind of them).

Let's get back to the ringing house phone. I picked up the phone and before I could say hello the voice on the other end said: "Hello, is that Mr Hyde?" I said "Yes," and the person responded by saying something that confused me "Mr Hyde I am a junior doctor from the local hospital, are you OK?" … "Err, fine thanks," I said. This didn't seem to satisfy him, so he asked again "No, Mr Hyde, I mean do you feel OK?" So, I told him that I'd just had a game of squash and I was just watching TV. He said "Squash?!...well…OK…Listen, Mr Hyde, I have just run the tests on the blood sample you submitted today. I am just ringing you to check that you are OK, because I have to go to another hospital and run some more tests and wanted to make sure that I spoke to you first. If you are indeed OK, I will phone you again in the morning once I have the full results." I tried to get him to tell me what he had found, but he refused to say anything and just said that he would discuss it with me tomorrow. Well, as far as I was concerned, that was a confirmation of my fears. Needless to say, we didn't have a good sleep.

The next morning I woke up as normal and for One second...One glorious second...Life was normal. I looked over at my beautiful wife and kissed her good morning and went into the bathroom. As soon as I looked in the mirror, the events of the previous night came flooding back. And with them came (what was to become a familiar feeling) a cold shiver, that rose up my back and engulfed my head. We went through the motions that morning, trying to act normal.

I made breakfast as usual and we had just sat down when the phone rang. It was the same doctor that I had talked to the previous night. He said that the results had come back and that I should pack some clothes and come into the hospital as soon as possible. I pressed him again on what was wrong with me and he refused to discuss it over the phone. He went on to say, "I think it's best if we discuss it face to face." I gave in and said "OK, where do I come?" There was a short pause and he said the "Cancer Ward"... The Cancer Ward...The Cancer Ward! He might as well have said the "You've got a week to live ward" or the "Don't pack more than a few days' worth of clothes because you won't need them ward" ...F*@k!... I put the phone down and turned to Debbie and told her what the doctor had said. We both burst into tears and hugged. Unfortunately, at that exact point our eldest daughter Rebecca, who was supposed to be away at University, walked in and said: "What's up?" We had decided not to tell either of our daughters anything until we had a definite diagnosis, but we hadn't planned on our eldest coming home unannounced. We had no choice but to tell her what had happened and where I was going. Obviously, there were tears, followed by a firm demand. She pleaded with me "Promise me that you're going to be OK?" She asked me to promise because as far as she was concerned, I never break my promises. So, I made the promise.

In a funny way, it gave me strength. I don't break my promises and I have just promised my daughter that I will be OK, therefore, I will be OK. You can't argue with that logic, can you? After calming Rebecca down, I packed a bag and I set off for the hospital with Debbie.

WoW: You don't have to bear the burden on your own, share your fears with a partner or a close friend.

Chapter 3

The hospital

The journey to the hospital was like...well...it was like travelling to the cancer ward of a hospital to see a doctor who specialises in the treatment of cancer, where you suspect that you are going to be told you have cancer...Sorry, I just can't think of a comparison that comes close.

As you might expect we were rather subdued and didn't say much, but every now and then Debbie would touch my hand and give it a little squeeze. I didn't feel scared or worried, I just felt numb. It was probably a wise decision for Debbie to drive us there, because I don't think I would have been able to concentrate properly on driving. Which, when I think about it now was a rather a selfish decision, because I can only imagine what was going through Debbie's mind. After all, she had just found out that her husband and best friend of 33 years, almost certainly had cancer. So, with hindsight, I should have insisted that we took a taxi to the hospital. Anyway, back to the car, where I was just staring blankly into the distance and thinking about nothing. I knew I was thinking about nothing, because I remember thinking about a relaxation class that Debbie had dragged me to. I remember that I was supposed to empty my mind and think about nothing. I remember thinking 'how can you possibly empty your mind and think of nothing?' But here I was, thinking of nothing. Which, when you think about it wasn't strictly true, because I was thinking about thinking of nothing.

I was dragged back to reality when the car came to a sudden halt. We had just joined the long and currently stationary queue for the hospital car park (apparently, a common issue with hospitals these days). We decided that it would be best if I got out and made my way to the 'Cancer Ward' on my own, while Debbie attempted to park the car. This is another decision I would change if I had my time over; because it wouldn't have made any difference if I had got to the ward 30 minutes later, but it would have made a significant difference having my best friend with me to hold my hand as I entered the hospital.

As I walked towards the entrance the numbness returned, but this time it felt more oppressive. It felt like someone had put plugs in my ears. I could hear muffled noises as I made my way to the huge glass double doors of the hospital entrance. *Those sliding doors would later become a symbol of my membership to an exclusive club that nobody wants to be a member of.* I could see a hive of activity through the doors, but I was still in a muffled state. As I got close, the doors automatically slid apart and a cacophony of sound hit me like someone had just ripped out my earplugs. There were people everywhere; doctors, nurses and porters crisscrossing the corridor with seemingly perfect precision. Patients in dressing gowns, some with drips connected to their arms, some with oxygen masks. Most of the patients were being supported by loved ones, except for one that caught my eye. She was sat on a bench with a nurse kneeling in front of her. The nurse was holding her hands and talking to her calmly and quietly. This image will stay with me forever; the woman touched her bald head and then looked up at the shop in front of her and started to cry...the shop was a wig shop. I had the sudden realisation that I would probably lose my hair. I hadn't thought about it before, because I'd convinced myself and I'd come to terms with the fact that I was going to die. I hadn't even thought about treatment! My mind was suddenly overloaded with random manic thoughts and the next thing I remember is trying to navigate the confusing array of signs in an attempt to find the cancer ward.

I couldn't remember what the ward was called, I couldn't remember the directions the doctor had given me over the phone. Debbie would remember, she was good at remembering directions, but she was still parking the car. The next thing I knew, I was walking through the entrance to the cancer ward. I made my way towards the reception desk, just as a young doctor was passing by. He stopped and walked over to me. "Mr Hyde?" he said while tilting his head to one side. I said "Yes?" He then approached me, shook my hand and went on to say, "We spoke on the phone? come with me." I followed him to an examination room where he proceeded to explain the situation in a very soothing and reassuring manner. At no point did he mention the 'C' word, and at no point did I really understand what he was saying. I may have looked in control of the situation and that I was not letting it overwhelm me. But the reality was, that my brain was a chaotic mess! My thoughts were bumping into each other and shouting "Oh shit! Oh Shit! Oh, Shit?'... Oh yes, I was in control.

The bits I remember were something about my white blood cell count being really high and my rigid stomach muscles were definitely not rigid muscles, but in fact a very enlarged spleen. He went on to explain that I had a defective chromosome and that he couldn't be 100% certain, but he thought I had a rare condition called CML (that wasn't the C-word I was expecting). If they confirmed it was CML, then it was something that they could treat. At some point during this explanation, Debbie came in to sit with me. In my mind I was thinking...'Great, I don't have cancer! What was I worried about?' He did a brief recap for Debbie, then gave me a leaflet to read while he went away to organise a bed and further tests. When he left the room, I looked down at the leaflet and that familiar cold shiver rose up the back of my neck and over my head and face. The leaflet said Chronic Myeloid Leukaemia! Shit!... I had Leukaemia! Sounds stupid when I think about it now, but that's what was going through my scrambled brain at the time. I gave the leaflet to Debbie and she started to read the important bits out aloud. I could see she was trying to be strong and hold back the tears, but occupying herself with reading the leaflet helped her focus.

She read out the symptoms that people normally experience if they have CML:

- Getting infections more often than usual... "Two urine infections and Three chest infections in the past twelve months...Me" I said
- Weight loss... "I lost twenty-five kilograms in twelve months...Me"
- Fatigue and looking pale... "Definitely Me"
- Abnormal bruising... "I have some amazing bruises...Me"
- Abdominal discomfort... "Me"
- Poor appetite... "Me"
- Sweating... "Me"
- Swollen painful joints... "Oh yes...Me"
- Headaches... "No... excellent...I can't have Leukaemia then!" I joked

After Debbie read each symptom out, we gave each other a knowing look. It's at this point that I felt let down by my old friend T'internet... He said I had stomach cancer and that my chances of survival were small, but it was quite obvious from the symptoms that I had Leukaemia!

Debbie was in the middle of telling me that I had a defective Philadelphia gene, when a nurse came in to take my blood pressure and weight. After taking my blood pressure he asked me to sit on a special chair with built-in scales so he could measure my weight. He said "Ninety-four kilograms" out aloud while writing on my hospital notes. Instantly all the stuff about cancer disappeared. I said, "How much?!" He repeated "Ninety-four kilograms." I gave him an astonished look and said, "Your scales must be wrong." He just laughed and left the ward. I worked hard to lose twenty-five kilograms...well...Me and my Leukaemia worked hard to lose twenty-five kilograms. I immediately turned to Debbie and shouted with a twinkle in my eye "I'll be buggered if some nurse with a pair of shitty scales is gonna add four kilograms to my weight!" She laughed in a way that said, 'you have just found out that you have leukaemia and all you're worried about is that some nurse has got your weight wrong?'

WoW: Firstly; you're not going to be able to take it all in, so don't try. Bring a loved one or a friend to the hospital. Secondly; put yourself in the hands of people who know what they're doing. The doctors and nurses do this every day, so let them do their job.

CHAPTER 4

If they say the bone marrow test won't hurt ... they're lying!

It wasn't long before the doctor came back. He said that my bed was ready and asked us to follow him to the ward where I would spend the next few days. It was more like a large room than a ward, with just two beds in it and the bathroom. Each bed was enclosed by curtains for privacy, so I couldn't see who my new roommate was. I sat down on the bed and Debbie sat on the chair next to it. We both listened to the doctor as he explained what was going to happen over the next few hours. I must admit that I wasn't really listening, because I was preoccupied with the dilemma of whether to change into my pyjamas or not. Don't laugh! It was really important to me at the time. The doctor then went away to organise all the important stuff that he had just told me about (whatever that was?). After he had left, I turned to Debbie and asked her "What did he say?" to which she answered, "Which bit?" and I said... "All of it" and then told her why I wasn't listening. She laughed and said, "What are you like?" She then went on to give me a very detailed account of what the doctor had said. Well...I think it was detailed, but I wasn't listening, because I still hadn't decided whether to change into my pyjamas or not. What? It's a very important decision to make. I can't just lie on the bed in my jeans, it just doesn't look right. Just as Debbie had finished filling me in, the doctor returned and said, "you can change into your pyjamas if you like" (dilemma over).

He went on to say that he needed to take some blood for yet more tests. "Do you have a preference for which arm I take it out of?" I said no, but in the days that followed my answer would change to "Whichever arm has the least bruising." He then said that they were just preparing the room for the bone marrow extraction. I turned to Debbie and said, "Who's having a bone marrow extraction?" She laughed and said, "You are! Weren't you listening?" Of course I wasn't listening! I had more important things on my mind.

He led us to a small examination room where a bubbly nurse greeted us and asked me to lie on the examination table and asked Debbie to sit on the chair next to me. She then continued with her preparation of a small table on wheels, which had various tools and medical equipment on it. The piece of equipment that caught my eye was a small electric drill with a rather long drill bit in it. The doctor explained that he needed to take a bone marrow sample and that it was a routine procedure and it didn't hurt. All the time he was talking to me, I could see the drill out of the corner of my eye. He presented me with a piece of paper and said that I would need to sign it before he could proceed. It basically said that I was happy for the procedure to go ahead and that I knew the dangers. I signed…what else was I going to do? He then pulled out another piece of paper and went on to explain that he would like to take "An extra sample for research purposes which would help in the…" I stopped him mid-sentence and said: "Of course." With the benefit of hindsight, I might have said "No!" Anyway, I signed the second sheet of paper.

While he prepared the equipment, the nurse asked me to roll on my side facing Debbie and to crunch up in the foetal position with my back facing the doctor. She went on to say that it was a routine procedure and that it didn't hurt. I should have suspected something at this point, but my mind was preoccupied. Debbie pulled up a chair next to me and held my hand. The nurse tried to talk to me and distract me from what was coming. However, she got on the topic of running, which interested Debbie more than me, so they were both quite happily chatting away just as the doctor said, "I'm just going to give you an injection to numb the pain."... Pain?...what pain!? I thought you said it wasn't going to hurt?! The doctor then said, "can you feel this?". To which I said "No", but before I could finish the 'o' in 'No' he started drilling into my hip bone. Which turned my "No" into a "Nougghhhhoooo!" The sensation was horrible! Every time he pushed and prodded there was shooting pain down my leg and a shudder up my spine. It was at this point I heard the nurse say, "Oh no, if I had to give a bone marrow sample I would ask to be put to sleep..." Put to sleep?... Put to sleep?!... *I thought you said it didn't hurt*!?

I had no idea how long this procedure should normally take. Although I did start to get the idea that this particular procedure was taking longer than normal when I kept spotting the nurse looking over to the doctor with a quizzical look on her face. It was obvious the doctor was having trouble drilling through my bone. I know this because he said so! The nurse and doctor exchanged one of those 'all-knowing' looks. 'You know, one of those looks that could not possibly be interpreted by any patient. The sort of look that means *'This isn't going to plan, and if I don't get through the bone soon, then I don't know what I'm going to do. For God sake keep the patient distracted.'* If that wasn't clear enough, he followed the look by whispering to the nurse that he was having trouble getting through the bone...no shit Sherlock!

As the nurse looked back at me her quizzical face changed

to a rather concerned face. She moved closer to me and said: "Let me hold your other hand." Apparently, I had been clawing my cheek with my free hand!

When the doctor had finally drilled through the outer layer of my bone, I was just on the verge of crushing the hands of the two delightful ladies next to me. Now came the weirdest sensation of all, as the doctor finally started to extract the precious bone marrow sample. It was the most weird and horrible sensation, a sensation that I can't describe. So, once it was over, my relief was obvious to all. I could feel the blood coming back to my face. I started to relax and talk to Debbie and the nurse, but inside I vowed never to let that happen again. Unfortunately, my relief was short-lived, because the doctor then said: "Now for the research sample…" '*No!*' I said…inside, and inside it stayed. Well, I couldn't really turn around and say that I didn't want to help research a cure for the very thing I had, just because I couldn't cope with a few minutes of pain…could I? I closed my eyes and braced myself to go through it all again.

WoW: If someone says a bone marrow extraction doesn't hurt…they're lying.

Chapter 5

You can take my pee, but you'll never have my poo

After the trauma of the 'simple painless bone marrow procedure,' we made our way back to my bed where I settled in to get some rest. A lovely nurse came around to introduce herself and explained that she would be my main contact throughout my treatment. She talked me through a 'starter' pack that she had given me, telling me what to expect in the coming days and weeks. She talked about the local cancer support group. I didn't see myself going to a support group. So, I told her that I felt OK and didn't think that I would need that sort of thing. Everyone was talking about 'after I get discharged', which gave me an amazing glimmer of hope. It was hope that there would be a future and I just wanted to start that future as soon as possible. I wanted to get out of there and back to normality. She smiled and said, "Of course, but the support is there if you need it." Debbie collected all the pamphlets and booklets that the nurse had left with us and started to read them. She came across a pamphlet that talked about defective Philadelphia chromosome which I apparently have. She went on to read that it is a mutation that occurs during the patient's life rather than being inherited. She said that it was unusual for someone of my age to get Leukaemia (Fifty years old). Apparently, you either get it when you are young or over sixty years old. Another reason for a defective Philadelphia chromosome is radiation damage, which made us

24

both raise an eyebrow because I have worked with radiation all my working life.

It was soon after this that the original doctor came back to see me and said that the results from the bone marrow wouldn't be back until tomorrow, but that he was ninety nine percent sure that I had Chronic Myeloid Leukaemia. He went on to say that he needed to get me on a course of broad-spectrum chemotherapy straight away to get my white blood cell count down. He had the tablets with him and some more forms for me to sign. Again, my ignorance showed, I thought, great! I'm on mild chemotherapy and not on the harsh radiation. Of course, I later found out that chemotherapy is a drug-based treatment and the radiation stuff is different treatment...that's why it's called radiotherapy.

I looked at the forms and he talked me through the list of side effects which included; hair loss, rashes, nausea, muscle and joint pains, etc. I signed, and my new companion 'the cold shiver' returned. Before the doctor left, he told me that I would have to drink at least 3 litres of water a day to flush out the toxins from the Chemo and that I was going to be monitored closely. Apparently, the surge of toxins could overload and damage my liver. I took the tablets and settled back to listen to Debbie reading out the detailed side effects that I may experience during my chemotherapy.

Thankfully another nurse came in and interrupted Debbie mid-sentence. She was pushing a trolley with a rather large number of disposable bedpans and urine bottles on it. She proceeded to put all the urine bottles on the cupboard next to me, 8 in all. Then she started to put the bedpans on the cupboard as well. She must have seen the puzzled look on my face and informed me that the chemotherapy drugs that I was taking are very toxic and that it was extremely important to analyse everything that comes out of my body. What she meant by everything was my urine and my poo. I looked at Debbie, then at the nurse, then back at Debbie, then back at the nurse and I said: "You are not having my poo." She smiled and said that it was important that they monitor my reaction to the chemo. I said, "You can have my wee, but there is no way you're having my poo." She laughed, with a look that said, 'We'll get your poo, they all give in eventually'. She then said, "you're going to have to go eventually," to which I responded, "I'm holding on to it until I leave the hospital." She laughed and shook her head knowingly. I thought 'She doesn't know me very well, I can guarantee you…she isn't getting my poo.' I heard her giggling as she left the ward. Debbie said things like "Don't be silly" and "They are just doing their job" and "It's for your own good," to which I said, "They ain't getting my poo and that's final."

With all that had happened that morning I was really starting to get tired. So I convinced Debbie to go home for the night and get some rest, which she reluctantly agreed to do. But before she did, she said that she would quickly pop down to the hospital shop downstairs and get me some snacks and drinks to get me through the evening. She wasn't gone long before she appeared with a bag of goodies. She smiled mischievously as she pulled a bottle of 'Lucozade' out of her bag and gave it to me. This won't mean much to you, but Lucozade was the cure-all from my childhood. Whenever I was ill, my mum would always give me Lucozade and said it would make me better and even now as an adult, I still subconsciously turn to it whenever I feel unwell. Next from the bag came a packet of favourite biscuits 'Jammy Dodgers.' Finally came a couple of packets of 'Monster Munch' crisps, another favourite from childhood. Debbie gave me a kiss and a long loving hug then left with tears in her eyes. I put my earphones on and settled down to get some well-earned sleep.

But before I could close my eyes, a nurse came in with a saline drip on a stand. She said that I needed to take the entire contents of the plastic bag to help me cope with the chemo. She then went on to insert a cannula into the vein on my left hand and hooked it up to the bag on the stand. She then quickly left the room and returned with the compulsory machine that goes 'beep'. She connected this machine to the drip and told me that it would beep every couple of seconds to indicate that the flow was good and that an alarm would go off if the flow was interrupted. She went on to say, "Try not to move your arm too much." Great! So much for getting some sleep! Every time I dozed off, I would roll on my side and the bloody alarm would go off and wake me up...this went on all night.

Then there was the water! I did as instructed and drank gallons of the stuff, which meant of course that I had to go to the toilet every fifteen minutes to relieve myself. Each trip to the toilet was pretty much the same: I would just be nodding off to sleep when the alarm on my cannula would go off and wake me up. I would then feel the need to go to the toilet. So, I would get up and start walking towards the toilet and then remember that I had to unplug the power supply from the drip, taking care not to bend my arm too much. Then, I would grab the stand with the drip on it and start to wheel it around the bed, only to remember that I had to get one of the disposable urine bottles. So, I would make my way around the other side of the bed to retrieve one of the bottles. All the time I was trying to be as quiet as possible so as not to wake my roommate. Once I had my bottle I would make my way to the toilet, do my business and repeat the whole process in reverse, only this time I had a disposable bottle full of pee. Every two or three trips I would press the button above my bed so that the nurse could retrieve a full bottle to take to the lab for tests. On one of my return trips, I tripped over one of my shoes and nearly dropped the bottle, but I managed to catch it before it spilt over the floor. But in the process, I bent my arm, which set off the alarm and woke up my neighbour. The rest of the return trips would end pretty much the same way: I would get to my bed, plug the power cord back into the drip, snuggle back into bed and try to get back to sleep. But, every time I was just about to doze off, the alarm would shriek and wake me up and the process would start all over again...and that was how it was all night. Until, that is, the drip finally ran out and the nurse came in to remove it and take it away.

Great I thought, I can finally settle down and get some sleep. It was at this point that the guy in the next bed started moaning. It started off as a slow and relatively quiet moan that soon became a more frustrated and much louder moan. He was moaning for at least thirty minutes before he rang the alarm to call the nurse. When the nurse came in, he told her that he wanted the drip that he was on removed. He said that it was causing him too much pain. The nurse said that he had to complete the dose of antibiotics contained within the drip, otherwise it would not get rid of the infection he had. She went on to say that if he could just last a couple of hours more, then they could take it out as planned. This did not appease him, he wanted "The damn thing out now!" The nurse said that she would have to get the doctor, because she couldn't make the decision to remove it. He then shouted, "Get the f*&king doctor, but you'd better be quick or I'm gonna rip this thing out myself!" The nurse went and ten minutes later a doctor came in and asked the guy in the bed next door in a thick

Indian accent "What seems to be the problem?" He went on to repeat his demand (in his thick African accent). He said, "I want this drip out now!" She obviously didn't understand him because she said: "You can't go on a trip...you are very ill and must stay in your bed." "No!" he shouted, "I want this drip out now!" She then repeated herself "You have to stay in your bed" I could tell this was driving him crazy. "No! ... I want this drip out!" he shouted back. I could tell she was confused, but she carried on with her stance and said "I know you want to go on a trip, but you can't even walk. You need to stay in bed." At this point, even I was getting annoyed, so I got out of bed and made my way around the curtains and said to the doctor "He wants you to remove the drip." She then looked at me as though I had just asked an inappropriate question and said quite angrily "He can't remove the drip! He needs to finish..." I interrupted her and said "I don't want you to take the drip out!...he does!... I don't even know him...I just want to get to sleep!" They went on to discuss the situation for the next five minutes and finally they came to a compromise...she took the drip out.

Great, I thought, I could finally get some sleep. I closed my eyes and snuggled into my pillow and was just slipping off to sleep when the lights came on and a trolley came clattering into the room "Breakfast!" I looked up at the annoyingly happy porter and asked him what the time was. "6:30 am" he said. I'm in hospital...Why on earth would I want to get up at 6:30 am? There didn't seem to be a choice in the matter, so breakfast it was. Just after I finished my breakfast Debbie came in with another bag full of goodies. It honestly felt like she had only been gone an hour or so. She asked me if I had managed to get any sleep, so I gave her the unabridged and fully animated rendition of my wonderfully restful night. She tried to be sympathetic, but it's hard to accept sympathy from someone when they are giggling. She had just composed herself enough to start showing me the contents of her goodie bag when the nurse came in. She checked my notes and then counted the bedpans and turned to me and asked: "You haven't used any of the bedpans?" I reminded her that there was no way I was going to poo into one of those things and that I was holding on to it until I left the hospital. I could see in her face for the first time that there was a realisation that I wasn't kidding. She shrugged her shoulders and said that my blood and wee would have to do.

WoW: Let them have your wee, but don't let them take your poo!

CHAPTER 6

How do you tell people that you have Lukemia...Leukemia...Leukaemia?

We decided not to tell anyone about my illness until we knew more about the diagnosis and the long-term outlook. The only exceptions were; our eldest daughter Rebecca, and Debbie's mum. Obviously, Rebecca knew because she walked in on us crying, so we had to tell her. We were supposed to be visiting Debbie's Mum and Dad in a couple of days, so Debbie confided in her mum and told her to keep it quiet until we knew more. Although the doctor said he was sure I had Leukaemia, he couldn't be 100% sure as to which type of leukaemia I had until the bone marrow test results came back. So, we planned to wait a little longer before telling our youngest daughter, Emma, who was away at university. We didn't want to worry her until we knew the long-term outlook. The trouble with plans is that they require people and events to follow them for everything to work properly.

This particular plan was thwarted by my dearest mother-in-law, who wanted to reach out to Rebecca, who she knew we had told. She wanted to let Rebecca know that she wasn't alone and that her grandmother was there to support her. So, she did what most people of a certain age would have done, especially if they had recently started using social media...she posted a message on Rebecca's Facebook page, saying that she was thinking of her in this difficult time. She thought that it was a private message and that only Rebecca would see it. Within minutes, Rebecca started getting messages from her friends asking her what was wrong. This was about 11 pm on my first night in the hospital and Debbie had just gone home. When I noticed the message, I immediately phoned Debbie and asked her to contact her mum to get the message removed. Although only a small number of people had seen the message, we decided that we had to tell Emma, quickly. And when I said we, I meant Debbie.

My mum had been unwell for some time and was in and out of the hospital, which meant that the whole family were really worried about her. So... when Debbie phoned Emma just before midnight, the first thing that came to Emma's mind was that her Nana was dead. So, before Debbie had a chance to explain why she was phoning, Emma asked: "Is Nana dead?" Naturally and instinctively Debbie said "No, it's your dad...," but before Debbie could finish the sentence, Emma burst into tears thinking that her dad was dead! You couldn't write this stuff, could you? Well...you could, but no one would believe you. Apparently, it took a while before Debbie could explain that Nana and her Dad were not dead. She went on to explain that I was in the hospital and that they thought I had Leukaemia and that I was going to be OK. I didn't know this had happened until Debbie came into the hospital the next day. Although I realise that it must have been a very traumatic event for Emma, it was almost inevitable that as Debbie told the story, that we would try...very unsuccessfully, to stop ourselves from laughing.

Looking back now, makes me wonder whether the doctors and nurses had ever heard so much laughter from one of their emergency wards before. I also wonder about my roommate behind the curtains, and whether the laughing was a good or bad thing? Did it lift his spirits or did it annoy him? That led me to wonder whether people expect the emergency cancer ward to be a solemn place full of fear, sorrow and pain? Or whether they expect it to be a place full of warmth, hope and humour. A place where people learn to deal with their condition and make the most of their time left, whether it be days' months or years. Then, I thought that if people see the emergency ward of a cancer hospital as a place of suffering, then perhaps they expect to suffer. Do they see other patients who set aside their suffering as somehow disrespectful to their fellow patients? As a kid, I saw hospitals as places where people went to die. It was the same as bungalows, they were definitely places that people lived in just before they died, and that's a fact. Well it is when you are ten years old. I guess what I am trying to say is that if you believe a place has no hope, then it won't. Fast forward to the present where my view on hospitals has changed dramatically. I now see them as places of hope and faith:

- Before you walk into a hospital you are full of fear
- When you walk in, there is hope
- When you put your life in the hands of the doctors and nurses...there is faith.

You don't have to be religious to have faith and hope.

After we had finished laughing, Debbie went on to say that some of our friends, who had also seen the post on Facebook, were asking what was going on. So reluctantly, we decided to start telling people. I asked Debbie to start with a phone call to my brother Chris, to ask him to tell my eldest brother Mike and sister Diane. She went outside to phone him and the conversation apparently started with her saying "Hi Chris, it's me, Debbie." It was very unusual for her to phone him so Chris was immediately concerned and said: "Hi...what's up?" Debbie said, "It's Tony he..." and then proceeded to blubber uncontrollably for fifteen minutes. From what I gather, as Emma did, Chris thought the worst and spent those emotional and I'm sure worrying minutes trying to calm my dear wife down just enough, so she could string a sentence together and tell him...'what the bloody hell was up!' I felt guilty asking Debbie to tell people, it must have been so emotionally draining, but there was no way I could tell anyone. What would I say? "Hi, it's Anthony...I've got cancer," of course I couldn't.

Well, there was one person I could and did phone, my oldest friend John. He had phoned me the previous year from his hospital bed to tell me that he'd just had an operation to remove a brain tumour. He was a fireman by profession and had spent his entire working life risking his own life to save others. It was such a shock when he phoned to tell me about the tumour, because just weeks before I'd had dinner with him and his wife Sue. We had a lovely evening chatting about old and new times. They told me of their plans to retire early and buy a house in the Lake District. Sue was a nurse and worked the night shifts. He also worked shifts, which meant they hardly got to see each other and were so looking forward to this idyllic retirement. Fast forward to that day when he was talking me through his diagnosis and the operation and his prospects for the future. While he was talking, all I could think of was the unbelievable injustice of it. Why him? He had just been saying how they had been saving for their retirement, they were looking forward to going on long walks and simply enjoying life together and now this. It's just not fair! Of course, life isn't fair, no one ever said it was. In the weeks after the phone call, I sent him a text every day with the corniest jokes I could find. Even then, I believed in the power of positive thinking and wanted to bring a smile to his face and let him know I was there for him. He lived a few hours away, so it would have been easy for me to pop in the car to see him, but he asked me not to and I respected his wishes. He said he felt like shit and couldn't concentrate and had to take frequent naps, so wouldn't be good company. I know now that I should have ignored his request and visited him, because just me being there would have given him someone to lean on and take a little bit of pressure off his family.

Anyway, fast forward again to my phone call to him. "Hi John, it's Anthony," I said. "'Allo...just a minute... I've got bad reception, I'll just walk in the other room...that's better, how are you doing?" he said. "Well, I know it's not a contest, but I think I've got you beat," I said. "What do you mean?" he said. "I'm lying in a hospital bed in the cancer ward." I went on to say, "I've got Leukaemia! But not just any old Leukaemia, they tell me I've got a rare form called CML - Chronic Myeloid Leukaemia." After a few minutes of disbelief and filling him in on the details, we eventually got to laughing and joking. There we were, two friends with life-threatening conditions, just laughing. A nurse came in to take my blood pressure, she looked at Debbie, raised an eyebrow and said that she would come back later. I'm sure a recently diagnosed cancer patient laughing uncontrollably must have been an unusual sight. Debbie kept looking at me during my telephone conversation. She kept shaking her head in disbelief that I was laughing so much. She said later "You didn't let him know how ill you really are." She went on to say "You have Leukaemia! Don't you get it? You could die!" The thing is, I did get it, I just didn't see any point in dwelling on it.

Then, there was my mum. We decided that there was no point in telling her that I was ill. She had advanced dementia and wouldn't have understood anything I or anyone else said. If, by some miracle she did understand, she would definitely have forgotten it by the next day. As I said in my introduction, one of the reasons for writing this book was to tell my loved ones the things that I couldn't possibly tell them at the time. So, if you don't mind, I want to say something to my mum. She died two years after I was diagnosed and I know that facing the possibility of my own death really helped me deal with her passing in a healthy way. I felt relief that her pain was over, I let go of any guilt I may have had over not visiting her more than I did. She knew that I loved her, just as I know that my kids love me. But I would still like to take this opportunity to tell her now about my illness. So, if you imagine that I am phoning her from my hospital bed, then this is how I think the conversation would have gone:

"Hi mum, how are you doing?"... "Good...Yes, I'm fine...well...there is one little thing"... "Now don't worry, I'm fine, but I've been to the hospital and they have told me that I have Leukaemia"... "It's a form of cancer, but don't worry, I'm fine, I promise."... "No, I can't have it cut out, it's not that sort of cancer, it's a cancer of the blood"... "No, it's not because I don't eat meat"... "No, it's not because I drank paint when I was a child"... "No! Of course it's not your fault."... "Yes, I've got clean underwear on"... "No, the girls won't catch it"... "Yes, I've got some Lucozade and buttercup syrup"... "Yes, I've had something to eat."... "Don't worry, I'll be fine, I promise...I love you too."

A year after my mother died, I lost my brother and dearest friend Chris. He had been ill for many years with heart and lung problems. But no matter how ill he was, he was always more concerned with my health than his. As soon as he found out that I had Leukaemia, he immediately volunteered to be a bone marrow donor along with his Son 'Little Chris' and my sister Diane (which brought me to tears when I found out). We used to joke on the phone about who was more ill. He was really pissed off when I told him that I had just had a pneumonia injection. That didn't last long, because within a couple of weeks he couldn't wait to ring me up and tell me that he actually had pneumonia. When he started to get really ill, at no point did I ever think that he would die...he was too young. We spent several days at his bedside knowing that he was near death. During those days there was a procession of his friends coming to say goodbye to a man they loved. It was so traumatic to watch but at the same time it also made me so proud. When it came to my turn to say goodbye...we all gathered around his bed and I held his hand and I spoke so beautifully and eloquently. Everyone was in tears, but just as I was getting to the really emotional finish, he slipped his free hand down to waist and gave his crotch a good scratch. Our tears of sadness were instantly replaced with tears of laughter. So even at the end he couldn't resist one last laugh.

My mother hadn't been herself for years and had been in pain for most of that time, so her passing came as almost a relief, which made it easier to deal with. It was so much harder to deal my brother's death, because he was taken before his time. Then I decided to take the same approach I took for my own situation. I looked at the love in his life and all the wonderful things he did and achieved. It made me so proud of him and also made me believe that he would have no regrets about leaving. I get sad when I think about him and every now and then I shed a tear, but I celebrate his life and I treasure being a part of it...and that really helps.

As with my mum, I would like to take this opportunity to be say a few words to him in the form of a letter...if you don't mind?:

"Chris, did I ever tell you that you were my dearest friend, and that I always thought you were a better version of me? You were so selfless, kind and loving. Everyone loved you. The only chink in your armour was your compulsion to cook naked (he never missed an opportunity to whip off his clothes). You bought me my first ever vinyl record, 'Don't bring me down' by ELO. That was the start of my lifelong love of music, so thank you. You also bought me my first new bike, which was the start of my lifelong love of fried food and beer….well, nobody's perfect.

You have always been there for me and I just wanted to say thank you. But before you go, I want to make you some promises, and you know that's a big thing, because I never break my promises. You were so worried about what would happen to Rosemary and the kids after you went…Don't worry… They'll be fine. But I promise to always be there for them, whenever they need me. Even when you were ill, you were more worried about me and my health, so I promise to stay healthy and to die old and of natural causes. I promise to raise a glass to you every Christmas, so that even my grandchildren to come will know of you and what a special person you were. And finally, I promise to at least once in my life…cook naked…Love you."

I included the sections on my mum and brother for two reasons:

The first and totally selfish one was to tell the world how much I love and miss them. The second was to show how I have dealt with their deaths in a healthy way. I wasn't consumed by grief, when I could so easily have been. I hope that telling you, may help.

The last thing I want to stress is that this period of my life has not been tragic or horrible. It has had some tragic and horrible periods, but overall my life is wonderful.

WoW: Make sure you fully understand what you have and what the prospects are before you start telling people, it will save any unnecessary heartache. And make sure you ban parents from commenting on Facebook!

Chapter 7

The Leukaemia Diet

I originally wanted to call this book the 'Leukaemia Diet' because of a funny theory that came to me regarding my dramatic weight loss. I've always had problems with my weight, but a few months before being diagnosed, I decided to make a last-ditch concerted effort to lose weight and regain the body I had in my twenties. When you look at the relationship between the mind and body, you inevitably think of it as a combination of the conscious and subconscious. Subconsciously the mind tells the heart to beat and the lungs to breath, consciously the mind tells the body to speak and walk, but why can't we consciously tell the body to burn more fat and lose weight or heal itself?

Which brings me on to my theory. What if, in my desperation, the message to lose weight managed to get through to my subconscious. What if, each major organ in my body had a basic consciousness and could communicate with each other on a base level, but the communication with the brain was problematic and complicated. I imagined an emergency meeting being convened by the main body committee, where the heart addressed the lungs, kidneys, liver, spleen, stomach and bowls...

"Now lads, I have just received an urgent message from the brain. He asked...nay...he pleaded with us to lose weight, apparently it's our last chance...Any ideas?"

I imagined a murmur from all the organs as they discussed

this unprecedented event. "What about if I refused to let any food in?" said the stomach.

"You know what happened last time you did that? We all suffered," said the heart.

"I could restrict the blood to one of the legs so it would eventually drop off, that would lose a lot of weight," said the blood veins.

"It's a good thought, but I think we're supposed to lose weight all over and not just in one place," said the heart.

Then the thyroid gland said, "I could go hyperactive... that...would..." Then he fell asleep, so that suggestion was ignored.

After much deliberation, the usually shy spleen said that with the help of bone marrow and all the blood cells he could enlarge himself and use up huge amounts of energy and burn huge amounts of fat and that would lose weight fast. It was voted on and passed with a majority (the thyroid gland was still asleep).

So, my body meant well and in the short term it had the desired effect. Unfortunately, it had a slight downside of giving me leukaemia. Who can say conclusively that this didn't happen on some level? I really wanted to lose weight...and I did. What I'm trying to say in this rather surreal chapter and will continue to say throughout this book, is that the power of the mind is something that we cannot underestimate. This is clearly evident for pharmaceutical companies who carry out drug trials; they have to take into account that potentially as much as thirty percent of the people in any trial will show an improvement in their condition due to the placebo effect. That means that three in ten people will get better because they believe they are taking a magic pill that will cure them. I know that this is probably based on drug trials for minor conditions and not life-threatening conditions, but it still shows the effect that positive thinking can have.

WoW: Don't underestimate the power of positive thinking. It has the power to replace despair with hope and help in the healing process.

Chapter 8

Leaving hospital

During my stay in the hospital, I hadn't given much thought to 'going home,' because for most of the time I thought I would never leave. So, imagine my surprise when the doctor came and sat on the edge of my bed with the results from the bone marrow test. And said that I did indeed have CML, but it was treatable and more importantly survivable. He went on to say that the latest bloods and urine tests were showing that I had responded really well to the Chemotherapy, and my white blood cells were coming down quickly. He mentioned another test result that would become the most important indicator of my leukaemia levels, and that was 'BCR-ABL.'

Apparently, when I was first admitted my BCR-ABL level was above 90%, but now he said that it was coming down dramatically. He said that if I wanted, I could finish the rest of chemotherapy treatment at home. It was as though I had been awoken from a daydream and been asked to come back to the real world. It was an unbelievable feeling and such a wonderful surprise. He said that I would have to come back into the hospital every few days to get my bloods taken and see how I was progressing, but he was happy for me to go home. He also mentioned the possibility that I may need a blood transfusion if my white blood cell count fell too low, but even that filled me with intensely positive emotions, because my youngest daughter Emma had just given blood for the first time. The thought that there was the tiniest possibility that I would be given some of my daughter's blood if I had a blood transfusion was mind-blowing.

While I was in my own little world, thinking about getting better and not dying. The doctor said something about organising my drugs with the pharmacy and filling in my discharge paperwork. He then did something that seemed to finalise the deal, something that said, 'OK Mr Hyde, you can leave now'...he shook my hand and said: "Well Mr Hyde, I'll say goodbye now." He got up and left, as though he had just fixed a problem with my computer. This man had been the one who phoned me late in the evening to ask if I was OK, after he had just got the results from my first blood tests. He was the same man who greeted me at the hospital the following morning. He was the man who was with me for the next few days and seemingly never slept. My wife said she saw him come into the hospital one morning. She said he just looked like a normal young man with a rucksack on one shoulder arriving at work. But his work was saving people's lives and he treated it as just another day at work. We should never let these people forget how much we appreciate what they do.

If there is one thing the NHS in the UK is brilliant at, it's handling emergencies. If you are in dire need, it's like a well-oiled machine. The doctors and nurses are so calm and efficient at such a frantic and traumatic time. They give you such confidence, that you immediately place your life in their hands without a second thought. So, if I had to give them a trip advisor review, it would be five stars for emergency response. But when you look at other areas of their business you soon realise that they are a victim of their own success. Every resident of the UK expects to have access to this amazing service, but unfortunately they are so understaffed and underfunded that they cannot give the same response to non-emergency cases. This means that as soon as you become one of these non-emergency cases, you can expect that well-oiled machine to get a bit sticky and slow. I soon found out that being told you could leave the hospital and actually leaving the hospital very rarely happen in close succession. I was all packed up and waiting to leave about 10 minutes after getting the good news from the doctor, but had to wait for the senior consultant before I could leave. Every time a nurse came by, we would ask when we could go and they would say each time that 'the consultant is nearly here.' Several long hours later, I was finally sitting in the car and we were making our way home…I couldn't believe it.

I was going home…I could actually start to think about the future. As soon as I knew I was going home there was one thought that consumed me and that was to get back to as normal a life as I could, as soon as possible. I also vowed to get fit and healthy again, so that night we had Fish'n'Chips and a glass of Prosecco…well…I was celebrating! I know what you're thinking, 'Prosecco and Chips' is so middle class! And I would have to respond by saying that my favourite meal and the one thing I was craving was Fish'n'Chips from the 'Chip Shop', but you can't celebrate not dying by having a beer. So, it had to be Prosecco. We had a lovely evening, just my wife and me chatting about what had just happened over the last few days. We also talked about the future and what we would love to do. I think it was at this point that the idea for this book was born. I went to bed early that night, mainly because I was extremely tired, but also because I was looking forward to sleeping in my own bed.

Instead of waking up the next day refreshed I actually felt fatigued and feeling almost like I had the flu. Notwithstanding my feeling like crap, I said to Debbie that I wanted to walk into town and back like we normally did at the weekends. She didn't think it was a good idea, but I convinced her that I felt fine and that we would take it nice and easy. And so, we did, but I must admit that I felt different, I felt weak and a little exposed. We managed to get into town without incident and then suddenly my hip just seemed to collapse on me and I couldn't walk properly. Now, let me emphasise that I was only fifty-one years old and not a fragile pensioner, so the hip issue came out of the blue. Debbie was worried and said we should get a taxi home. Of course, I said no and said that I could walk it off. Which I did and we eventually went to one of our favourite coffee shops and had a coffee and a guilt-free slice of cake. Guilt-free in the sense that I had lost so much weight over the last few months that I felt good about myself. Suitably refreshed and nourished it was time to return home. Debbie asked again about taking a taxi home, but I said I was fine, and I was...sort of. The walk home would normally have taken about 40 minutes at a leisurely pace. On that day, however, we were walking more at a snail's pace, so I expected it to take a little longer. The difference in pace was highlighted most alarmingly when we realised that we had been walking for about sixty minutes and were only just past the halfway mark! Shit, I thought to myself...I was knackered and really wasn't sure I could make it home. Debbie was concerned, so we had a rest so I could recharge my batteries. But the problem was, I continued to get more and more tired even as I sat there supposedly 'recharging my batteries.' So, I lied and said I was ready to set off again because I thought if we don't move now, then I would most likely collapse into a heap. ninety minutes after leaving town I found myself shouting at the sky "Who the fuck moved the house?" I just couldn't believe that we weren't home yet. I was getting slower and slower; my muscles were on fire and I thought I would never make it home. Debbie was really concerned, but we couldn't get a taxi now because we were walking down narrow lanes, so we had no alternative but to carry on. After what seemed like an eternity we finally made it through the front door. I had just enough energy to make it upstairs, where I collapsed in a heap on the bed and slept for the rest of the afternoon. The positive thing to take from this was that I'd broken the donkey's back and subsequent walks got easier. If I had any advice to give to people in the same situation it would be to take the first couple of days easy because your body is fighting the battle of its life, so give it a bit of slack and build up the exercise slowly.

This episode showed me that things were going to be different from now on. I knew I was on chemo, but I also knew that after the chemo I would be on long term medication for the foreseeable future. My body wasn't the same and I knew I now had to listen to it and try not to overdo things. Now that didn't mean that I could put my feet up and take it easy!... No, I was determined to get fit and to do that, I had to get used to my new 'base level.' What was my 'new base' level? Well, it consisted of aching and sometimes painful joints, aching and sometimes painful-burning muscles, continual and sometimes severe fatigue, and let's not forget the horrendous muscle cramps. The old me would not go to the gym or go for a walk if he had aches and pains like this, but the new me couldn't afford to because if I did, then I would never go out. I knew I had to treat these aches and pains as nothing unusual, they would have to be put away in a cupboard and ignored... Easy. ☺

WoW: Take things easy when you start chemo, your body is fighting a battle and needs all the help it can get...plenty of rest,

water and good food...just take it easy.

CHAPTER 9

The sunset still looks the same and a flower is still a flower

When I started writing this book I always envisaged that it would be read not only by people with cancer but also by their family and friends. I hoped that I could let fellow sufferers know that they are not alone and that life does not have to be bleak and depressing. I also hoped that I could give their family and friends, an insight into what their loved ones might be going through.

I know it's difficult to know what to say to someone with cancer, so I am not poking fun, but when you are on the receiving end, it really can be quite funny. What do people say? Well the most common things are: "I bet you appreciate every bit of your life now" ... "I guess it changes your priorities" ... "I bet you notice things that we take for granted, like sunsets and the beauty of nature?" ... "I bet you're going to live life to the full now?"

The truth is, I already appreciated my life. I knew what the most important things in my life were and that's my family and friends. So, sunsets are the same now as they were before and a flower is still a flower. This appreciation for what is important in life started about fifteen years prior to being diagnosed with CML. I was analysing our household spending, because I just couldn't figure out how we had no money at the end of each month, even though we both earned a decent wage. While looking through the bank and credit card statements I noticed that my dear wife had managed to spend £3,000 with Costa Coffee (other coffee shops are available)! And that was just the spending I could track via credit cards. I had no idea how much she had spent in cash. In her defence, she would normally have our two daughters as her partners in crime and there would usually be cake involved. I started to think about the amount of money that was being spent on just one thing, and a question came to me. So, I turned to Debbie and asked, "Do you remember any of those visits to Costa Coffee?" and she looked a bit puzzled and said, "What do you mean?" I just simply asked whether any of those visits were memorable. She thought about it and eventually said: "No, Why?" I said that she had spent £3,000+ on something that she couldn't remember, and asked whether it would be better to spend that money on a holiday that we could remember? Now you're probably thinking that she stopped going to Costa Coffee and we used the money to go on lovely holidays? Well, that's not quite what happened, it was more fundamental than that. We rarely went on holiday; we hardly ever celebrated our wedding anniversary. We just lived a good life, enjoying good food and good wine with family and friends. After that day, we decided that we would start doing memorable things, starting with holidays. When I say memorable, I mean just that, not a simple off the shelf beach holiday. I would arrange holidays that were/are different/unique/beautiful and above all, fun. Whether it is a luxury weekend in London, a peaceful stay in a lighthouse in Ireland or camping near Stonehenge, they had to be memorable.

One of my favourites was a family road trip through Italy. Where me, my wife, our two children and my precious but ever so slightly unreliable Alfa Romeo 159 drove from the North of Italy down to the Amalfi coast. There were two main themes to the holiday; the first was to take my Alfa to the Vatican to get it blessed by the Pope and the second was to track down and visit my uncle, who I had never met before. I spent many months working out the itinerary; we initially drove to Dusseldorf where we took the car train to Munich, which was real fun. When we got to Munich, we spent a lovely evening with old friends who were living there and in the morning we drove over the dolomites to lake Garda. I had booked rooms in a farmhouse on the mountain overlooking the lake. It looked easy to get there on the map, but the reality was oh so different. The road to the farmhouse started out as a normal country road, then as we started to climb the mountain it started to turn into a single-track road that got narrower and narrower. Eventually the road disappeared and we were driving on what can only be described as a wide footpath with 2-metre-high hedges either side. At one point it got so narrow that I had to pull my wing mirrors in because they were touching the side walls! We inched our way along this dirt track all the time praying that we didn't meet another car coming the other way (we have a photograph of my wife standing in the middle of this dirt track with her arms spread out and almost touching the side walls). Eventually and with great relief we emerged from the dirt track to the wide-open field on which we could see the farmhouse. The owner came out to meet us and was amazed and puzzled as to how and why we could have possible driven down the footpath to the farm! After all most people drove in through the main entrance from the rather wide main road. Once we had all stopped laughing he showed us where we would be staying for the next couple of days, and on the way let us pick some fresh figs from a series of fig trees lining the foot path. During our stay we visited Verona and Venice, then we drove down through Italy stopping at Bologna, Florence,

Perugia, Rome and the Amalfi coast. We would spend a couple of days in each place and enjoy the local sites, food and drink. We thoroughly enjoyed each stage of the trip, but as we got closer to Rome the thing that started as a bit of a joke turned into a real thing. I started to seriously think about getting my car blessed by the pope. So when we were outside the Vatican I stopped a passing Nun and asked her where I had to go to get my car blessed by the Pope. She gave me such an astonished and definitely disapproving look and walked off without a word. Instead of putting me off, it gave me the incentive to carry on. After the third unhelpful Nun, I decided that Nuns weren't going to help in my quest. When we got into the Vatican courtyard I asked one of the Vatican guards to direct me to the car blessing area, but I soon discovered that the Vatican guards talked less than the Nuns! I was just about to give up when I spotted an old priest who looked kind and approachable. I stopped him and said, "Excuse me father, but could you tell me where I go to get my car blessed by the pope?" He looked at me and smiled, then he thought for a while and eventually said "Well my son, do you see the gift shop across the square?" he pointed to a small building across the square. "Well, each cross in the gift shop has been blessed by the Pope"... "So, if you buy one of these crosses and place it in your car, then you can say that your car has been blessed by the Pope"... "And all for a very reasonable price" he said. He looked me in the eyes, touched my shoulder, then winked and walked off into the crowded square. I thought to myself ... 'Wow, that has got to be the coolest priest I have ever met.' I went to the gift shop as instructed and purchased a small wooden cross and put it in my car...job done!

Prior to starting this holiday I had written a letter to my uncle to say that I would be coming to Italy with my family and that we would love to see him. I didn't get a reply, but I had hoped that he would phone me at some point during the holiday. By the time we had got down to the Amalfi Coast I had given up on my uncle making contact, so was overjoyed and a little bit nervous to finally get a phone call from him. Between his very limited English and my limited Italian we agreed a time to meet the next day. I knew from my mother that my uncle was very ill and had just come out of hospital where he'd just had a quadruple heart bypass. It made this visit so important, as I couldn't be sure if I'd ever get another chance to see him. My sister had also driven to Italy on her own road trip, so we all met up in a small village called Liberi in the mountains overlooking Naples. It was one of the most memorable days of my life, spending time with a whole section of my extended family that I had never met before and to finally meet my uncle Attilio. We all sat around a table eating, drinking and laughing. Looking back its hard to believe how much fun we had even with the language barrier. It had a very emotional end to the day when my uncle looked around the table surrounded by his family and said, "I can die happy now" and within a month he did. Wonderful and precious memories

I have always had a dream that if I ever won the lottery I would buy a lighthouse big enough to live in. It would have big F*&k off walls surrounding it and possibly a jetty with a boat. Debbie has always humoured me with this particular dream, but as we have got older she started to get concerned that it might become a reality. So in a bid to put me off the idea she organised a holiday in a lighthouse in Ireland. It had five floors, two bedrooms, a cosy living room and a kitchen on the top floor. Debbie thought that spending four days walking up and down stones stairs would put me off the idea of living in a lighthouse. The reality was that it backfired on her, because we had an amazing time and after the second day Debbie confessed that she loved it. We spent the days going for walks, reading, writing (this book) and just being with each other.

I shared these memories not to 'show off', but to 'show you' that I had already had an epiphany about the quality of my life and what and who was important. I valued my life, my family and friends. So when I thought I was going to die and I looked at my life and I wasn't filled with regret and unfulfilled dreams. I saw a life full of love, loved ones and wonderful memories. Knowing this gave me such a warm reassuring feeling, so much so that the dread and fear seemed to slide away. So, if you are reading this book after finding out your future is far from certain, then go out and enjoy life as much as you can, while you can. If you are reading this book and you are fit and healthy, then... go out and enjoy life as much as you can, while you can.

WoW: I'm not gonna say live every day as though it was your last because that's just unrealistic. What I am saying is appreciate what you have and what is precious to you...and I mean really appreciate it...then enjoy yourself and create memories!

CHAPTER 10

It's not just you going through this

As the 'sufferer' it's perfectly understandable to forget that it's not just you going through this because your loved ones will be suffering too. They will be just as terrified as you are and will feel utterly helpless. They will feel that they don't have the right to hurt because this is happening to you and not them. But the truth is that this is happening to all of you and all of you are hurting. They will attempt to be strong for you, especially when you are at your lowest and most in need. They will try to be loving, comforting, helpful, constructive, inspiring and strong. This is exactly what you need in those first few days because you won't be thinking straight or taking things in properly. You may think you are, but you won't be. Everyone needs someone to support them through this difficult time. I was lucky in that I had a network of family and friends who were only too willing to be there for me. I was extra lucky because I had my wife. The fact that she was my best friend as well meant that she was a one-stop-shop for comfort, love, inspiration and strength. She would do all the information gathering and leaflet reading and I would just ask for the verbal summary, leaving me to focus on me. If you're not fortunate to have close family and friends, then there are always support groups only too happy to welcome you, and the cancer nurse assigned to you will give you their details.

Having said all that, I think that relying totally on your support group should only be a short-term thing. I emphasise 'I think' because I'm no guru, I am just speaking as a well-meaning fellow sufferer. I encourage you to use this support group to get through the tough early stages, then I believe you need to take ownership of the situation. One of the best ways of doing that is to turn your attention to your loved ones. They were strong for you and now you need to be strong for them, comfort them and reassure them. I focused initially on my wife. She had seen her strong and independent husband break down in tears and confess that he was scared and she did what I expected her to do and that was to be brave, braver than I have ever seen her before. I could tell that she was terrified, but she was always calm, comforting and encouraging. There was no way she could have kept that up for long, so as soon as I was in control again, I took that weight off her shoulders. She could then let go and finally break down in front of me. I couldn't take away her fear, but I could make her forget about it for a while and bring a smile to her face. As for my daughters, that was trickier because their dad was and is indestructible. There are no sensible words of advice I can offer here because I did not think logically. I operated on pure emotion with my kids. If I was supposed to be indestructible in their eyes, then I'd bloody well better be indestructible. Just as I promised Rebecca before I went to the hospital, I had to promise Emma that I would be OK and I wouldn't die. Even that illogical and emotional commitment to my daughters gave me strength. Being strong for others really does help you to be strong. When you're going through something like this, you need all the positive energy you can get.

WoW: Lean on your loved ones so you can become strong enough to repay them by allowing them to lean on you.

CHAPTER 11

Every song on the radio is about death and your bald friends want you to lose your hair

If there is one thing I can guarantee you when you or anyone close to you first gets diagnosed with cancer, it's that every song on the radio will suddenly be about death and loss. Every interview on the radio or TV is about cancer or death or dealing with the loss of a loved one. I noticed this on my first morning at home after leaving the hospital. The sun was shining through the patio doors, the table was beautifully set with delightful things to eat for a very special breakfast with my darling wife. All was good, I turn on the radio and a record from my childhood is playing. 'Seasons in the Sun' by Terry Jacks with those classic lyrics "Goodbye to you my trusted friend." I looked over to my wife who seemed oblivious to the meaning of the song and I felt a wave of emotion sweep over me. After I had managed to get my way through that emotional song I was then presented with 'Gone too Soon' by Daughtry. At which point the wave of emotion subsided and I began to think that someone was winding me up. The very next song up was by 'Duran Duran' and I thought thank God for that! A happy song. It was their hit 'Ordinary Day.' Have you ever listened to the lyrics? Just listen to the bit where Simon Le Bon sings "Where is my friend when I need you most? Gone away" I just turned to my wife and said "what the hell is going on…is this for real?... I haven't heard one happy song yet." I got up and switched station. There was an interview in progress where a celebrity was talking about the loss of her husband to cancer. I just turned to Debbie and said: "Oh for God's sake!" This stuff can go one of two ways, it can bring you down to a dark place where you dwell on the negative or it can make you laugh. As I'm sure you will have guessed by now...I laughed.

I remembered while at the hospital, my CML nurse had talked about the support groups I could contact to help me through this difficult time. I immediately said that I was OK, and I was. I felt strong, my mind was in a good place and anyway I was lucky to have my own support group, my family and friends. I hadn't seen any of my friends since being diagnosed and I knew that they had contacted Debbie to ask if they could come and see me, so rather than have a procession of visitors at home we decided to arrange a get together at a local pub for breakfast. I was a little nervous about how the morning would go, so I thought if I was nervous what would they be feeling? I'm sure they were wondering what I looked like and what they should say and wondering if it was going to be awkward. I didn't want any of that, so I made sure that I was upbeat and let them know that I was OK and that I was still the same person I was before. I was self-deprecating with regards to the Leukaemia and encouraged them to join in (they didn't need much encouragement). I told them the whole story of how it all started (pretty much the whole of this book) and we laughed and had a great time. I was so happy that I had such wonderful friends...I felt loved and very lucky indeed

It's funny, how little people know about Leukaemia (myself included), but even I knew it was life-threatening cancer. One of my dearest friends who was there at the breakfast meeting didn't even know that much, and his wife took pleasure in telling the group how he wasn't too concerned about me when he first found out that I had Leukaemia. She was initially surprised by his reaction, but then realised he didn't quite grasp the severity of the situation. She asked him what he thought Leukaemia was? to which he replied "it's an infection, isn't it?... I guess he'll be on strong antibiotics for a while?" She chuckled to herself and then went on to explain to him what leukaemia was and how fortunate I was to still be around. It was at this point that he finally grasped the severity of the situation. I won't mention Dan's name because I don't want to embarrass him, but his knowledge of Leukaemia didn't stop there...oh no....when he knew that we were all getting together he asked his wife (who is a nurse) "Is it catching?" Dan is lucky that I haven't mentioned him by name!

Then we come to my follically challenged friends who were a little disappointed to see that I hadn't lost my hair! They were even more disgruntled to hear that I was, in fact, getting extra hair growth...you just can't please some people! We were very loud that morning, the combination of funny stories and feelings of relief resulted in the volume control being turned up to 11. I was aware that people who were close by may have thought that our behaviour and what we were joking about was perhaps inappropriate, but we were not being disrespectful in any way. I didn't want my friends to worry about me and I certainly didn't want them to treat me differently. I made sure that our first meeting was full of laughs and was as normal as possible (under the circumstances).

WoW: Don't get paranoid, you will notice things more...and yes...all the songs on the radio are about death when you're dying, just as they are about failed relationships when you have just broken up with your partner...Try and see the funny side.

CHAPTER 12

The side effects

It's funny when you think about the dangers we have come to accept in our daily lives. I'm thinking specifically about our blind ignorance or disregard of the potential side effects when taking any form of medication. It could be a simple 'over the counter' painkiller or a prescribed antibiotic or even the contraceptive pill. They all come with a leaflet containing a long list of side effects and invariably we will take these drugs without even reading the leaflet. We seem to have a blind faith that these drugs will do their job and that nothing bad will happen. I guess we all think that the chances of succumbing to one of the long list of side effects is negligible and in most cases we would be correct.

Unfortunately, in my experience it's not quite the same with chemotherapy. Even though the list of side effects presented is much shorter (or at least the list that they showed me in the hospital was short), I can pretty much guarantee that you will get several if not all of these side effects at some point during the time that you are on them. I can also guarantee that you'll end up attributing every ailment, ache and pain that you have to them as well.

I remember when I was taking the broad-spectrum chemo tablets. I had to visit the hospital regularly to have my bloods taken, see the doctor and be examined. These visits had become something of a routine. I'd get to the hospital over an hour before my appointment, just to make sure I could get a car park space. Then I would generally start with a cup of coffee and a piece of cake in the hospital cafe, which was right next to the hospital entrance. It was one of those cafes run by volunteers, so I soon learnt not to expect too much in terms of speedy service, which was fine because I would rarely be in a rush. After picking up my coffee and cake, I would find a secluded table and just sit quietly and people watch. After looking around for a few minutes I would invariably look over to the hospital entrance and think back to when I first came through those double doors. I would relive the emotions as though it had just happened; the fear, the helplessness and the utter loneliness. Inevitably my eyes would fill up with tears. I never had to worry about the people around me and what they would think, because I knew that we were all in the same boat. We were all members of that exclusive club that no one really wants to be a member of. All of us had our own encounter with death, either directly or indirectly and we were all doing our best to cope. So, there was no need to feel embarrassed, because I knew that everyone else in that cafe at some point had shed their fair share of tears.

After finishing my coffee and cake, I'd dry my eyes and then slowly make my way to the cancer outpatients waiting room. Once there, I would take a ticket from the wall dispenser, sit down and wait to get my bloods taken. During those first 6 months I had so much blood taken by so many different nurses that I began to recognise the different types of nurses working in a hospital. First, there are the student nurses who are generally nervous, but are warm and kind. Unfortunately they make the process of taking blood a painful one. Leaving you with the biggest and most colourful bruises. Then there are the experienced, but cynical nurses, who perhaps look at nursing as just a job and perform their duties efficiently, but with little or no warmth. They take your blood quickly, but can still make it painful and leave you with nearly as much bruising as the student nurses. Finally, there are my favourites, the 'vocation' nurses. This is not just a job for them, they became nurses because they wanted to help and care for people. They are so gentle and warm, they know that you are most likely scared and possibly in pain, so they will go out of their way to take your mind off it for a precious few minutes. They take blood painlessly and leave no bruising... "Remember to put pressure on the plaster for a few minutes to stop the bruising" ...beautiful people.

After giving blood I would then queue up at the main reception desk, hand in my appointment sheet and ask, "How long is the delay in appointments today?" and the receptionist would almost always say "oh...there's no delay at the moment." We both knew that there would be a delay of anything from one to four hours! I found that the best way to cope with this long delay is to remember that this hospital and these people had saved my life and they are continuing to keep me alive. It would be very ungrateful of me to complain now. It wouldn't be so bad if I could just put on my earphones and listen to music. Unfortunately, if I did I wouldn't be able to hear the nurses when they came into the waiting area to call out my name. In reality, even listening very carefully for your name in my hospital wasn't a guarantee that you would hear your name either. There was one adorable Caribbean nurse who was always there when I went for my appointments, but her command of the English language was...how shall I put it? at best, a close approximation. When I first saw her, she came into the waiting area looking at a medical card in her hand and all the patients in the waiting room were on tenterhooks leaning forward and cupping hands over their ears (the average age of the waiting room was probably 65). I wondered what was going on, until she spoke, then it all became clear. She looked down again at the medical card, then looked up and shouted "Sanon Fipak!" ... she paused expectantly and looked around the waiting room for Sanon to stand up... "Sanon Fipak!" she shouted again...no one stood up. She shrugged her shoulders and went back to the examination rooms. A few minutes later she came out again with a fresh medical card and shouted, "Tree Hard!" ... "Tree Hard!?" Lots of people were looking around and whispering urgently to each other, but no one stood up. The nurse was now starting to get annoyed and turned to a fellow nurse and said, "None of my patients have turned up". She came back later to try again to see if Sanon had turned up yet. Again she shouted, "Sanon Fipak!"... "Sanon Fipak!?", with frustration in her face she turned to go back to the examination rooms, but as she did, a lady stood up and asked, "Do you mean Sharon Fitzpatrick?" and the nurse said "Yes! I've been calling you for ages...come with me". I later found out that Tree Hard was Trevor Howard. This gave me good preparation for when she eventually called out my name. She came out flushed with success of finally getting Sanon and shouted "Anyon Hiddi!" ... "Anyon Hiddi!?" ... So I immediately stood up and said, "Do you mean Anthony Hyde?" to which she said, "Why is everyone asking me what I mean?" I smiled and said that it was hard to hear clearly in the large waiting room, then followed her to be weighed. Of course, my friends never quite believed me when I told them, so I recorded her on several occasions to prove that I wasn't making it up. She has become a bit of a legend in my circle of friends.

Anyway, back to this particular visit. I went through to see the doctor and he asked how I was getting on with the chemo drugs. I told him that I was coping OK, and that the side effects were manageable, mainly because I was still off work and could rest and take things easy. He said that I had responded really well to the chemo and that there would be no need to have a blood transfusion, which was a relief. He then talked me through the next stage of my treatment. He talked about TKIs (Tyrosine Kinase Inhibitors), which are targeted chemotherapy drugs that target just the mutated/cancerous blood cells and not the healthy ones (unlike the broad-spectrum chemo drugs that are indiscriminate). He said that I would probably be on this drug for the rest of my life, which had shocked me. I thought that CML was treatable, I assumed that I would get to some point of full remission and that would be it. I never thought that I would be living with leukaemia for the rest of my life. My mind then went into dream mode, where I imagined that I would be the wonder patient who made an amazing recovery and would be off the drugs in six months. This is not necessarily a bad way of thinking because it pumps you up and puts you in a positive frame of mind. The down side is that when two years have passed and you are still on them, then it can be a little bit disheartening. So, my advice would be to think more along the lines of "I am going to get back to a normal life" because that is a more achievable goal. The doctor went on to say that there were three main drugs I could take. The first was the original Leukaemia drug Imatinib (Glevec), it came in the form of a single tablet that would only need to be taken once a day and he went through a list of side effects, including nausea, edema (swelling of the face, feet, hands), muscle cramps, bone pain, diarrhoea, haemorrhages, skin rashes, fever and of course hair loss (you can't have a list of side effects without hair loss, it just wouldn't be right). The other two drugs were more complicated to take. If I remember correctly they had a tablet that had to be taken twice a day, but they couldn't be taken within two hours of eating. The side effects were similar, but there was an additional emphasis on heart and lung strain. He did say that if I didn't get on with the one I chose, then it would be easy to switch. I didn't need much time to decide. I thought that since I had asthma and a family history of heart problems I would go for the tried and tested Imatinib option, which also seemed less hassle with just one tablet a day. I had found the side effects from the chemo fairly easy to cope with, so I thought that things would be similar with the TKI... It was a nice thought, but I would soon find that life would be very different with this drug.

I stopped the broad-spectrum chemo drugs immediately and started taking Imatinib. For the first few days after switching to Imatinib I felt fine, but then I started to get more and more fatigued. My muscles and joints started to ache and at times were painful. After a week or so I would wake up each morning feeling as though I had the flu, but without the runny nose and sore throat. As the weeks went by the joints and muscle aches and pains and the flu symptoms became the norm. This new norm would be joined occasionally by severe cramps and when I say severe, I mean severe. The first episode happened while I was fast asleep in bed one night, when I was suddenly wrenched from a deep sleep with the most excruciating pain in my leg. I instinctively jumped out of bed and tried to get my leg in a position to relieve the cramp, but every position I chose caused further cramp in a different part of my leg. It was agony, and after 5 minutes of this I started to suspect that this was not a normal cramp. It was at this point I remembered something the nurse said at the hospital. She said that the drugs would strip me of vitamins like calcium, potassium and magnesium. She said I should probably take supplements and make sure I had a balanced diet and always have a banana handy. She also said to drink plenty of water to flush out the toxins and that would also help with the fatigue. So, I quickly made my way downstairs (in agony), where I hurriedly grabbed and consumed a banana, then drank a large glass of water along with a couple of pain relief tablets. The cramp carried on for the next 20 minutes or so, it was so painful! Eventually it calmed down enough for me to get back to sleep, but in the morning, it felt as though someone had taken a baseball bat to my leg. It was so sore and uncomfortable; I could hardly walk on it. So, from that day on I made sure that I took supplements and drank plenty of water, well, more water than I used to drink. I still have problems with cramp, but I have never had a severe cramp episode like that one.

I thought it might be useful to go through the side effects that I have experienced and what I have done to alleviate them:

Cramp

The cramps were initially, extremely painful and would last far longer than a normal cramp episode. My pre-emptive approach is to take vitamin supplements of Calcium, Potassium and Magnesium and of course drink plenty of water (two-three Litres per day). An isotonic sports drink also does the trick. My cramps are still regular, but not so painful and very manageable. I know that putting my arms and legs in certain positions will bring on cramp, so I can avoid it most of the time. When I do get a bad episode of cramp I have discovered that rubbing in magnesium oil really helps, whether it's the act of massaging the muscles or the oil itself I can't be sure. All I know is that it works for me.

Joint and muscle aches and pains

I live with a low-level ache in both my joints and muscles, which on occasion rises to moderate pain. When the pain gets bad I often use an anti-inflammatory cream or tablets, which does help, but doesn't take away the discomfort completely. If I am honest with myself, as time goes on I can't decide which aches and pains are a result of the drugs and which are a result of normal age related wear and tear.

Fatigue

Fatigue is something I am always aware of, but try not to let it affect my life too much. I have found that drinking plenty of water regularly throughout the day helps, as does good healthy eating (lots of veg, pulses and fruit). I find that regular snacking throughout the day is better for me than 3 big meals. I also know that exercise plays a very big role in fighting my fatigue. It took me a while to discover that if I took things easy and rested to alleviate my fatigue, then the opposite effect would happen. Instead of feeling refreshed the next day, I actually became more fatigued. So, I decided that the only way forward for me was to arrange a regular game of squash with a friend, mainly so I couldn't back out. Although it was initially very difficult, I soon got into it and afterwards I felt so good. I found the more I exercise I did, the less I felt fatigued. Don't get me wrong, I was knackered after any exercise session, but it was a 'good' knackered. You can tell the difference between being worn out from exercise and being fatigued. If you are anything like me, you will grow to love the feeling of being worn out from exercise, it feels very rewarding.

Swelling, Bloating and Stomach Aches

I probably experience bloating once or twice a week and it

generally results in my face, hands, stomach and knees swelling significantly. With the swelling of the hands, stomach and knees comes discomfort, for example my hands swell so much that I cannot make a fist properly. Although my face is affected during a swelling episode and my cheeks look very puffy, my eyelids are pretty much swollen all the time. I can get some relief from the swelling by taking powerful diuretics prescribed by the doctor, they never seem to help my face swelling.

My stomach is often bloated and it is hard to determine whether it's a direct result of the medication or a change in my body since developing Leukaemia. Whatever the reason it is always uncomfortable and occasionally becomes painful. I haven't yet found a reliable remedy for this one yet, other than not eating large meals.

Vomiting

Every three to six months I tend to get a new batch of Imatinib from a different manufacturer and although they are supposed to have the same ingredients, they do often have a slightly different construction. The best ones are individually packaged so you can tear off an individually packaged tablet and put it in your pocket just in case you need it. These tablets are also film coated, which means you can swallow them without water if you have to and they do not taste of anything. The worst would come in a foil package and do not have any coating, so you can taste the tablet, which can be disgusting. It is these tablets that would end up making me vomit and feel sick. So, I asked my CML nurse to put on my notes that I should only have film coated tablets.

Skin complaints

When I started chemotherapy, my skin became very dry all over my body with my lips suffering the worst. I used a general moisturiser for my body and a chap stick for my lips, both of which helped greatly. Later, with the TKI the dry skin went back to normal and was replaced with a sensitive scalp. There would be a few sore areas and a couple of regions where the skin appeared to get thicker like a scab. If I scratched this area the skin would come away leaving a very sore area. I have been experimenting with ex-foliating scrubs to remove the excessive skin and then applying a vitamin E oil...currently this approach appears to be alleviating the symptoms slightly.

Burst blood vessels

This is a weird one and I am not sure whether it is attributable to the drugs or not. I have seen a couple of posts from sufferers on the leukaemia Facebook page that I follow, where they have had similar episodes. So, I will mention it just in case you are unlucky enough to experience it. About a couple of months after starting on Imatinib, I was sat having my breakfast when my left index finger and thumb started to swell. In a matter of 10-15 seconds they had almost doubled in size and after about 1 minute that area of my hand started to go a lovely shade of blue. It was very disturbing the first time it happened because I had never experienced anything like it before, so had no idea what was going on or when it would stop. I immediately ran my hand under cold water which seemed to help, but applying pressure seemed to work best. This has happened about five times over a two-year period and has always been located on my hands. When I told the doctor on one of my hospital visits, she said "Weird..." and went on to talk about other things (which made me chuckle inside).

Taste

Another strange thing that affects a lot of people taking medication for Leukaemia, is the way it can change your taste buds. It is very common for food and drink that used to taste wonderful, to now taste bitter and disgusting. For me the things that changed were beer and broccoli, both of which I loved and both of which tasted bitter after I started Imatinib. These taste anomalies usually go back to normal, for me it took about twelve months.

WoW: To help with cramp and fatigue take supplements like potassium (or bananas), calcium and magnesium (for the evenings magnesium oil massaged into problem areas really helps) and drink plenty of water (two litres a day).

Chapter 13

Free prescriptions for life...as long as you don't live too long!

There are people who say you should always look on the brighter side of life and other people who say a chapter should contain more than 1000 words…. well…this chapter is going to challenge both those statements.

When Debbie was reading one of the many pamphlets that we were given at the hospital, she came across an interesting paragraph which stated, "If you are being treated for cancer you are entitled to apply for free medical prescriptions for life." Well, this was a very small silver lining in a very nasty storm cloud, but never the less a silver lining it was. So, without further ado, I emailed my CML nurse and asked her whether I was eligible and if so, how did I go about applying. She promptly said that she would get the form filled in and sent out to me. She said that all I had to do was sign the form and send it off. This would save me quite a bit of money because I had to pay for my Asthma inhalers and blood pressure tablets each month, so it was well worth doing. Within a week, the form came as promised and I duly signed it and posted it as instructed. The form said that the decision would be made in one or two weeks and if successful, the medical exemption card would be sent out within a week or so. I would bore people with how I was going to get free prescriptions for life… "For life!" I would say. I felt as though I was in an exclusive club. After all, I was going to get free prescriptions…for life!

It was about three weeks later when I received the card. We were having breakfast at the time, so when I returned with the letter held high I said proudly… "Free prescriptions for life." Debbie and my daughters were all getting bored of this by now, so were not that interested. Regardless of their apathy I opened the letter to find my medical exemption card, which I held aloft saying "free pres…." I stopped midstream, which suddenly got my family's attention. "What's wrong, Dad?" said Rebecca. I started to laugh. I had looked at the details on the card and apparently my free prescriptions for life card…only lasted five years… *five years!* What did they know that I didn't?

WoW: You are entitled to free prescriptions while undergoing treatment for Leukaemia and that includes TKIs like Imatinib.

CHAPTER 14

Back to work

Initially, the hospital signed me off work for two months, which at the time I thought was far too long. My immediate thought was that I'd probably lose my job and that at my age I would struggle to get another one. I know now that this wouldn't have happened because my employer was very good with me. I also know now that cancer survivors have certain rights in the UK, so it's worth reading up on them if you think your employer is not being fair.

Anyway, I was off and felt quite good, so I decided not to waste this time and decided to go on long walks every day and started doing various jobs around the house (those ones that I always meant to do, but had never got around to doing). By the second week my activity tracker said that I was the most active person in my town. I had also redecorated the kitchen and built a table and chair set for the garden. By the third week I was ready to go back to work, not because I was a workaholic or that I was bored of being at home. I just felt ready and wanted to get back to normality as quickly as possible. I'd gone from making my peace with the fact that I was going to die, to thinking about my future. I was elated and just wanted the Leukaemia to take a back seat and my life to get started again.

As I said, I was convinced that my Leukaemia would be undetectable in record time and the doctors would be amazed at my recovery, so would recommend that I came off the Imatinib. So, on one of my regular visits to the hospital I asked the doctor if I could go back to work early and although he was a little surprised, he had no objections and agreed. I thought that when my employer heard that I wanted to come back to work they would be happy, but in fact he was a little surprised. They were concerned about whether I was ready to return to work so soon after chemotherapy. I assured them that I felt fine and that I wanted to come back full time as soon as possible. They agreed, only if I supplied them with a letter from the hospital to say that they approved. Simple…or so I thought! I asked the doctor at the hospital for the letter and he said he would get one sent out to me within the week. After that first week passed and the letter hadn't come, I contacted my CML nurse and she said that she would push the doctor to get it sorted for me. Another week passed and still no letter, but as I had a regular appointment at the hospital coming up I decided to ask again then. As it turned out he had the letter waiting for me when I arrived and he apologised for the delay. He then went on to explain why it had taken so long. Apparently, the letter was written on the day that I asked for it, but it then had to be emailed to a secretarial service in India, where they proof read it and typed it out on to official letter headed paper and posted it back to the doctor. The doctor then checked the letter and found there were a couple of errors, so he amended them and sent the letter back to be reprinted. This whole process took three weeks! He said that apparently, it was cheaper to do it this way than to have a dedicated secretarial service in the hospital!

Finally, my first day back at work came and I must admit I felt very weird walking in after so long away. Inevitably I spent the whole day answering questions and did absolutely no work. Everyone wanted to know about my Leukaemia… "What was it?" … "How did you get it?" … "Did you have chemo?" …

"How come you've still got your hair?" … "So, is it gone now?" It was lovely to see so many genuinely concerned people. The first few days were great, it was just what I needed, getting back to normality. By the second week I must admit that the side effects from the Imatinib really started to make their presence known. I started to get really exhausted, my joints and muscles would ache and were occasionally quite painful. My exhaustion was compounded by the fact that I had to get up at 5:45am each morning and travel sixty minutes by car to get to work, then do a full day of work before travelling sixty to eighty minutes back home. On retrospect, it would have been wiser to phase my return, perhaps starting with just a couple of days a week for a while until my body got back into the rhythm. After all, my working day was long and exhausting enough without having leukaemia.

WoW: You can definitely regain your previous life…just don't rush it, take your time and phase your return.

CHAPTER 15

Getting to know your new body (If you snooze you lose)

Having come to terms with the fact that you are likely to be on TKIs for the foreseeable future, it is then important to get to know your new body and what it can and more crucially what it can't do. I must stress that I am speaking from my own experience here because I know that there is a huge variation in how people react to their own TKI treatment and this ranges from people leading a perfectly normal life with hardly any side effects to people who suffer depression because they can't cope with the continual pain and discomfort.

Initially, I felt great because I had lost loads of weight and was moving around the squash court quicker than I'd ever done before. As time went on I started to have the odd bad day where I would wake up feeling really bad. All my muscles and joints would ache, I felt bloated and utterly exhausted and the thought of getting out of bed filled me with dread. I would still drag myself from the cosy duvet and go for a shower and shave, then off to work. Bearing in mind that I would start the day exhausted, you can imagine that the last thing on my mind when I got home was go to the gym or do any form of exercise. Inevitably, I started to put the weight back on, which in turn made me feel worse. It didn't matter what I did, the weight just kept creeping up. I couldn't understand it because even when I starved myself I still put on weight. That's probably an exaggeration, but not by much! There was definitely a change in my body because things that would have resulted in me losing weight before the Leukaemia did not work now, which was so disheartening and extremely frustrating. To make matters worse, the doctor told me that I would have to keep my weight down because the long-term exposure to Imatinib was shown to put pressure on the heart and lungs. Great! That's all I needed to hear.

I reached my lowest point about eighteen months after first being diagnosed. I would come home from work so exhausted that I had to go straight to bed for a quick twenty to thirty-minute nap, then I would cook a meal for my wife and a snack for me (because I was suffering again with acid reflux, so big meals in the evening were a no no). I would then sit in front of my laptop or the TV and vegetate for the rest of the evening. In the past I would always have a DIY project on the go, so would be doing things in the evenings and weekends. But I just didn't have the energy or inclination now. During the really bad days I thought that resting would help, but all it seemed to do was make it worse. This came to a head one evening when I looked at myself in the mirror and said, "Enough is enough I can't go on like this anymore." So that night I decided that I had to push through this because resting wasn't helping. So, I phoned up a friend and organised a regular game of squash in the belief that if someone else was waiting for me to turn up, then instead of vegetating in front of the TV I would drag my poor old body to the squash court. The first session was the hardest because I really didn't think I had the energy to pick up a racket, never mind play a full game. But as soon as I started playing I felt the fatigue slowly recede and I started to feel energised. After the game I felt great, I was so happy to have pulled myself from my usual evening huddle. Unfortunately, the next day I must admit that I was so stiff I could hardly move. As the weeks went by my energy levels went up and the chronic fatigue subsided to just fatigue. My body was still stiff after a game of squash, but that was a small price to pay. I felt as though I had more energy and started to become my old self again (not all the time…there were and are still bad days). It wasn't long before I started my DIY projects again, although I had to accept that I couldn't work as I did before. In the past for example; I could paint a room in an evening, but now it would take me two or three evenings, which was fine with me. I would just take my time, after all this was far better than the alternative of sitting in front of the TV every night.

The next thing to address was my diet. I was fasting for long periods of time, then when I did eat I generally ended up eating lots. Breakfast was my only safe meal of the day. I felt like I could eat anything without wondering whether I would be sick or worse…wake up choking in the middle of the night. So, I would indulge myself at breakfast and have things like fresh bread, croissants, cheeses, hash browns, eggs (fried and boiled), fried mushrooms, baked beans etc.…I would eat until I was full and it would last me all day. I would probably have a snack in the early evening. This often left me vulnerable to an energy slump, that was when I had a real depletion in energy and vitamins like potassium, magnesium and calcium. When this happened, feeling tired was the least of my problems because I would leave myself open to painful cramps. This cramp would sometimes appear in the most unusual of places. The most unusual and difficult to deal with was in my rib area. There would be no position you can get in that would alleviate it, so depending on where I was when this happened, I would have a banana or the isotonic drink. If I was home I would use the magnesium oil. As well as exercise, I needed to address my diet and find a program that will suit my leukaemia and associated issues.

WoW: You need to work through the pain and do regular exercise otherwise you'll be in danger of going into a downward spiral and end up in a bad place with a poor quality of life.

CHAPTER 16

Healthy eating/healthy lifestyle

Pushing your body to exercise when it really doesn't want to, is just a small part of getting better. You also need to consider what you're fuelling your body with. For example: The more foods I eat that are rich in potassium, calcium and magnesium, the less problems I have with cramp. So, if you can see a tangible result like that, then it's not such a stretch of the imagination to believe that other foods could have similar beneficial effects. Let's also not discount the psychological aspect; if I eat healthily, I feel healthy and if I feel healthy, then perhaps I am healthy? You'll soon learn (as I have) to accept all the help you can get...well almost. It does have to have a thread of logic to it. I'm not the sort of person who will buy healing rocks from Papua New Guinea on the recommendation of Gloria from work because she said it cured her really bad case of influenza. She slept with the rocks on her stomach and after 3 weeks the influenza was miraculously gone! And before you ask, there was no Gloria from work, but you get what I mean?

Just as I have learnt to ignore my body when it says it can't do any exercise, I have also learnt to listen very carefully to it where eating is concerned. I think it was about six months before my diagnosis, that I realised my body's relationship with food began to change. For example, if I eat lots of bread, I get bloated and feel really uncomfortable (but not all the time). Eating foods fried in certain types of oil makes me feel sick (but not all the time), and so on. I'm not saying that all these food reactions are as a direct result of the Leukaemia or the medication. I'm just saying they exist for me and they affect my life. I must learn to live with them in the same way I do with all the side effects. The frustrating thing is that the various food reactions that I experience are not consistent. This is not surprising when you consider that Imatinib can also cause stomach problems, which can take the form of stomach pains or aches. Some people complain of exaggerated effects from TKIs if taken without food, others say the same if taken with food! So, in my case the combination of a low-level intolerance for certain foods may be exaggerated by the side effects of my TKI... maybe? There were many occasions where I would be eating a meal and have a strong feeling that I would regret it, but I would still carry on and finish it, because that's what I was taught to do as a kid! And sure enough, I would indeed regret it afterwards, whether it was because of bloating, stomach aches or nausea. If you are anything like me, then you must learn listen to that very quiet voice inside, it knows what it's talking about.

Eventually, I came to my senses and decided to listen to that little voice. I cut down or stopped eating the foods that really disagreed with me and started to look at healthy replacements, but I needed help. So, I turned to my trusty friend, T'internet. We hadn't talked for a while, ever since I ignored him when he said I should see a doctor about my urine infection…and then about my rigid stomach. So, I sat down with my laptop and started to research healthy eating for cancer sufferers. As expected, I found lots of advice ranging from common sense to frankly, rather weird. The common-sense advice came from websites like the Macmillan Cancer Support website, which said that being overweight increases the risk of getting cancer and encouraged eating a well-balanced diet during and after cancer treatment. They also mentioned that 'eating more fruit and vegetables can reduce the risk of certain cancers.' The World Health Organisation said we should incorporate in our diet 'a minimum of 400g of fruit and vegetables per day for the prevention of chronic diseases such as heart disease, cancer, diabetes and obesity.' The Medical News Today website had a really interesting article entitled 'Tips for a healthy immune system.' It gave a lot of useful information about the immune system, how it works, what can affect it and how to boost it. The article reaffirms that consuming a healthy diet and regular exercise will help your immune system function properly. It goes on to say that lack of sleep can reduce the effectiveness of the immune system, so getting a good night's sleep is very important. They also said stress can reduce the effectiveness of the immune system and that "the anticipation of a happy or funny event increased levels of endorphins and other hormones that induce a state of relaxation" ...which in my book means humour is good for your immune system!

What about the rather weird websites? Well, I couldn't get copyright permission to share what they advised, so I'll leave you to discover them for yourself.

To summarise ... surprise, surprise! ... it's nothing new, it's just common sense. Eat a well-balanced diet with lots of fruit and vegetables, drink lots of water, not so much alcohol, keep fit, try and keep the weight down, get a good night's sleep and have fun.

WOW: There are times when you need to ignore what your body is telling you and then there are times when you really need to listen to it

Chapter 17

It's my Leukaemia

I thought long and hard before including this chapter, because even I must admit that some of my inner thoughts might be best left exactly where they are. The thought that someone might be comforted to know that they're not weird and someone else thinks like they do, changed my mind. That doesn't however, take away the risk that nobody else thinks like me and anyone reading this will think that I am a very strange person indeed. My wife would say "Nothing new there."

As I've said previously, I have never seen my leukaemia as a disease. I don't see it as an injustice. I don't see it as a punishment. I don't see it as an unwanted intruder. From the beginning I personalised it, by always referring to it as 'My Leukaemia'. That meant that I couldn't and cannot stand it when people say, "You're going to beat this cancer." Why would I want to beat myself? And another thing, have they never watched the movies? Anytime one of the main characters is mortally injured and the co-star says, "You're gonna be OK and you're gonna beat this... *dead!*" ...you know he's going to die!...*so don't say it!*

I approached my condition in a slightly different way. I decided to come to a mutually beneficial agreement with my leukaemia; he *could stay as long as he let me lead a normal life.* Sounds strange I know, but somehow it felt right for me. This approach enabled me to remain positive throughout my illness, because...I guess I was never fighting anything...it was more about getting to know my new body? I have also tried to be as normal as possible with my loved ones and friends, and lead that 'Normal' life. When people ask, "How can you stay so positive?" I usually tell them that at no point did I blame my leukaemia. I go on to say that my leukaemia has brought out the best in me. If you think about it, my leukaemia hasn't really caused me that much pain. Most of the pain and discomfort I has been due to the side effects from the TKI drugs.

Now comes the really strange stuff. If I am honest with myself, having leukaemia makes me feel special. "I have Chronic Myeloid Leukaemia"... It's a talking point...and if I am really honest with myself...I would miss it if it were gone. I can hear many of you saying, "This guy is nuts!" But perhaps there are a few of you saying nothing, because maybe you feel the same? I'm not a masochist, I don't enjoy the pain. I don't enjoy the discomfort, but I do enjoy the fact that I have found the power and strength inside me to overcome huge obstacles and that makes me feel proud of myself.

Don't get me wrong, if a doctor came offered me a magic tablet that could cure me, I would jump at the chance. What I'm trying to describe to you is my relationship with 'My leukaemia. I have talked to people with similar or worse conditions than me. In a lot of cases there were feelings of injustice and anger, which went on to consume them and in turn made their suffering worse. All I could see was them getting into a downward spiral to despair and depression. Looking back, I can see that my approach meant that at no point was I angry at the injustice of it all, which in turn gave me a really healthy foundation for what was to come.

Another thing that I have seen Leukaemia sufferers get hung up on, is the fact that to the outside world we look OK. I have read articles and blogs where sufferers talk about their anger towards people who think they are OK because they don't show the pain outwardly. They go on to say that they are suffering in silence and people should be aware of it. Whereas I always wanted to give out an image that I was OK, because I didn't want people to worry or be uncomfortable around me. So putting a sign on my head to inform everyone that I have leukaemia never really appealed to me. If, as a leukaemia sufferer, you get worked up because people don't treat you like you have a life-threatening disease, then perhaps you should look more to yourself than others. I know some of us really suffer both physically and mentally, but the last thing you need to do is add to it. I could be wrong, but I suspect the people who get upset that their leukaemia isn't acknowledged, want to be pitied. Whereas, I look for admiration, which I feel puts you in a much healthier frame of mind. I get on with my life and try to do all the things I did before. I love it when someone finds out that I have leukaemia and they are amazed that I am carrying on as normal. This makes me proud and gives me an extra bit of positivity, which in turn gives me a little extra boost.

WoW: Try not to think that what is happening to you is a gross injustice, a punishment or some form of victimisation for past wrongs. Try to own it... after all, its your body and your cells that have mutated, so personalise it. It's your leukaemia or cancer and you should make the most of your current situation and don't concentrate on asking why this happened.

CHAPTER 18

Passions for life

I have lots of passions: my family, friends, music, painting, photography, gardening, DIY...and one that seems to link them all together...cooking. I feel that the key to coping and recovering from any illness is to have a passion. I happen to have lots of passions, but all you need is one. It's something to look forward to, something to get out of bed for. When people ask me how I feel, the best way to describe it is, like waking up every day with the flu, but without the runny nose. So, then they ask, "how do you manage to get out of bed each day?" My answer is 'baby steps.' Each day I don't think about how I am going to make it to work when I feel like Shit. I just take baby steps. I just sit on the edge of my bed and contemplate whether I can stand up and I invariably do. Before I know it I'm in the bathroom, where I sit (yes...I said sit) and read the news headlines on the phone, then I shave and shower. I make my way down to the kitchen where I make my breakfast and sit quietly for fifteen minutes. I take a cup of tea up to the bathroom ready for when Debbie wakes up. I dress and before I know it, I'm in the car and on my way to work. Yes, I have a strong will, but if I didn't have things to look forward to, then I don't think I would have the incentive to do what I do. You're now asking yourself, how come he manages to summon up the energy to get up to work every day when he doesn't list 'work' as one of his passions? Well, I do love my job, but it isn't one of my passions. I have always seen it as enabler for my passions and for that I am eternally grateful. So, that's why I am willing to drag myself out of bed every morning without complaint.

I believe that passions inspire, encourage and heal. The power of the mind is something not to be underestimated and I don't. My mother was Italian and she raised four children on her own in a country where she couldn't speak the language very well. She was strong, selfless, independent, resourceful, stubborn …and a bit of a nutter. Everything she did was for her family, her passion was her family and that passion gave her the strength to get up each morning and work hard all day to put food on the table for her children (even when that meant that sometimes she went without). I was born in Stockport, England and soon learnt the phrase: An Englishman's home is his castle, but from my mother I learnt that an Italian's castle is his family. I share the same passion for family that my mother had and I hope I have passed this on to my children. With that passion for family comes the passion for food and for creating and sharing food with friends and loved ones. To this end, I even built a pizza oven in my garden so we could have pizza parties (and we have had lots of them!). Now, I'm not saying you should go out and build a pizza oven, but what I am trying to say is that you should find out what you are passionate about and celebrate it. A passion should be something to look forward to, something you can share with family and friends, but above all, something that makes you feel good. So, I've changed my mind... yes... go and build yourself a pizza oven!

Of course, I didn't stop at the pizza oven, or the handmade pizzas, because I needed somewhere for family and friends to sit down and eat together. Now you're really going to hate me for this...I decided to build a simple table and chair set, and when I mean simple, I mean big! I've lost count of the number of wonderful evenings we have had sat around this table. Good food and good company is good for the soul and in turn is good for the body. Now, I'm not saying you need to go out and build a big table and chair set, especially not when you're undergoing high dose chemotherapy like I was, but then again...why not? Go ahead and build a table and chair set! Just take it easy.

I could have stayed in bed while going through chemotherapy, but something inside of me just wouldn't lie down. I was full of the joy of life and all I could think about was getting back to normality. I also wanted to stay positive, because I thought that I had a better chance of surviving if my mind was in a good place. After building the table and chairs, I decided to redecorate the kitchen, after the kitchen I attacked the garden, and then I started writing this book...What will you do?

WoW: Everyone needs passion in their life...and the more passion you have...the more life you have.

WORDS OF WISDOM

The biggest and most helpful words of wisdom I can share with you, is to face and come to terms with the possibility that you might die. Once you have done this, you'll find that your whole outlook changes and you can cope with just about anything.

1 - If you think something is wrong with you...do not open your laptop...see the doctor and don't put it off. I was lucky, but my CML could have progressed to a stage that was not easily treated and I could easily have died. I also could have ruptured my spleen...and died.

2 - You don't have to bear the burden on your own, share your fears with a partner or a close friend.

3 - Firstly; you're not going to be able to take it all in, so don't try. Bring a loved one or a friend to the hospital. Secondly; put yourself in the hands of people who know what they're doing. The doctors and nurses do this every day, so let them do their job.

4 - If someone says a bone marrow extraction doesn't hurt...they're lying.

5 - Let them have your wee, but don't let them take your poo!

6 - Make sure you fully understand what you have and what the prospects are before you start telling people, it will save any unnecessary heartache. And make sure you ban parents from commenting on Facebook!

7 - Don't underestimate the power of positive thinking. It has the power to replace despair with hope and help in the healing process.

8 - Take things easy when you start chemo, your body is fighting a battle and needs all the help it can get...plenty of rest, water and good food...just take it easy.

9 - I'm not gonna say live every day as though it was your last because that's just unrealistic What I am saying is appreciate what you have and what is precious to you...and I mean really appreciate it...then enjoy yourself and create memories!

10 - Lean on your loved ones so you can become strong enough to repay them by allowing them to lean on you.

11 - Don't get paranoid, you will notice things more...and yes...all the songs on the radio are about death when you're dying, just as they are about failed relationships when you have just broken up with your partner...Try and see the funny side.

12 - To help with cramp and fatigue take supplements like potassium (or bananas), calcium and magnesium (for the evenings magnesium oil massaged into problem areas really helps) and drink plenty of water (2 litres a day).

13 - You are entitled to free prescriptions while undergoing treatment for Leukaemia and that includes TKIs like Imatinib.

14 - You can definitely regain your previous life...just don't rush it, take your time and phase your return.

15 - You need to work through the pain and do regular exercise otherwise you'll be in danger of going into a downward spiral and end up in a bad place with a poor quality of life.

16 - There are times when you need to ignore what your body is telling you and then there are times when you really need to listen to it.

17 - Try not to think that what is happening to you is a gross injustice, a punishment or some form of victimisation for past wrongs. Try to own it...after all its your body and your cells that have mutated, so personalise it. It's your leukaemia or cancer and you should make the most of your current situation and don't concentrate on asking why this happened.

18 - You need to work through the pain and do regular exercise otherwise you'll be in danger of going into a downward spiral and end up in a bad place with a poor quality of life.

19 - Everyone needs passion in their life...and the more passion you have...the more life you have.

ACKNOWLEDGEMENTS

If I could only thank one person, it would be my wife Debbie. It is for her that I drag myself out of bed each day. It is for her that I cope with all the pain and discomfort. She is my strength and my reason for living. To my daughters Rebecca and Emma you have been so brave and make me so proud. To my mum and brother Chris, I miss you so much. You were always there for me. To my sister Diane and brother Mike, thank you for your love and support. To my oldest friend John, thank you for our 'same old custard' chats over the phone. To my Witney brigade; Dan, Sarah, Bill, Sue, Mark, Tracey, Peter, Marie, Wendy, Donna and Jonny......To Rosemary, Little Chris, Katie, Tom, Katie, Nat, Zeppie, Christina, JuJu, Sam, Luke Ginette, Mary, Anthony, Adam and the rest of my Manchester and Blackpool family....to Reg &Vera, Simon...to the Poole brigade (of which there are hundreds)...to Sue & Adrian and Sue W thank you for all your love and support. To my employer and colleagues at Oxford Instruments, thank you for all your support and understanding. Finally, and most importantly, to all the doctors and nurses who have helped and continue to help save my life...thank you just doesn't seem enough, so to you I promise that I will do something significant with the extra time you have given me...and you know I never break my promises.

Appendix

Some helpful facts on leukaemia

I thought it would be useful to pull together some information on Leukaemia in what I hope is an easily digestible format...so here goes:

What is Leukaemia?

Leukaemia is a blood cancer. Its where your bone marrow produces defective/mutated white blood cells that never mature and do not perform the job they were designed for. If untreated, this ever-increasing number of mutated white blood cells will eventually cause organ failure.

Types of Leukaemia

There are four main types of leukaemia:

- Acute Myeloid Leukaemia (AML)
- Chronic Myeloid Leukaemia (CML)
- Acute Lymphocytic Leukaemia (ALL)
- Chronic Lymphocytic Leukaemia (CLL)

The Acute versions are fast growing and the Chronic ones are slower growing. My doctor said it was very important to determine which type of leukaemia I had, because that would determine which treatment I would need and also what my outlook would be. In fact, he wasn't 100% sure until he got the results of the bone marrow test back.

Phases of CML

I was told that CML develops slowly and has three phases:

- Chronic phase.
- Accelerated phase.
- Blast phase.

Chronic phase

Most people diagnosed in this stage may have no symptoms and they can have the leukaemia controlled with tablets...no being rushed into hospital for chemotherapy!

Accelerated phase

If the Leukaemia hasn't been spotted early or treatment has been ineffective, it can progress to the accelerated phase. In this phase, there are more blast cells in the blood or bone marrow (less than 10%). And of course with this phase comes a whole host of symptoms that I have detailed earlier in the book, such as:

- Tiredness
- weight loss
- bone pain
- Sweating

Note: Blast cells are the defective/mutated blood cells.

Blast phase

Again, if untreated or treatment has been ineffective the leukaemia may progress to the accelerated phase. In this phase, more than 20% of the blood cells in the blood or bone marrow are blast cells. Needless to say, this stage is not good place to be.

Chemotherapy for blood cancer

Leukaemia is very sensitive to chemotherapy, so depending on the severity of the condition when diagnosed, patients may or may not receive a course of chemotherapy. I significant number of patients in the accelerated and blast phases of CML will have chemo at some point in their treatment.

How does Chemotherapy work?

Chemotherapy drugs work by damaging cancer cells ability to divide which in turn stops the cancer from growing.

Most chemotherapy drugs are delivered through the blood stream. This means they can reach cancer cells anywhere in the body.

Why chemotherapy causes side effects

Unfortunately, chemotherapy drugs also affect healthy cells in your body. Some of the main areas affected by chemotherapy are areas where new cells are being made at a high rate. This includes:

- bone marrow (where blood cells are made)
- hair follicles
- digestive system
- lining of your mouth.
- Hence why people often feel sick or lose hair.

Sex

I was advised that unprotected sex while undergoing chemotherapy was a no no, because the chemotherapy drug could be transferred to my wife. This wasn't too much of problem for me, because I was either very tired or feeling nauseous during that period.

Legal Stuff

The most important thing to remember is that if you have cancer in the UK there are laws to protect you from being unfairly treated at work.

Reference Sites

www.macmillan.org.uk 'This information was produced by Macmillan Cancer Support and is reused with permission.'
www.who.int
www.medicalnewstoday.com

MORE FROM THE AUTHOR

The Mamma Nero Diaries

The Mamma Nero Diaries is a son's tribute to his mother, and her unsung journey from war-torn and poverty-stricken Italy to the cobbled streets of Manchester. The Diaries are full of humorous stories, as seen through a son's eyes. They describe a life of great hardship and sacrifice, but also of courage, principles, humour and hope... a hope that tomorrow would be better.

Anthony's mother taught him so many things. She taught him that if a pigeon with a ring around its ankle lands in your backyard it means God wants you to make a pie tonight. She taught him that if people come to visit, you should feed them – even if it means you go hungry the next day... and when they leave, you give them any remaining food you have *and* some of your plates and cups as a parting gift. She taught him that the best way to end an argument was to smash all the plates and cups that were left over from the last lot of people who came to visit... She also taught him to buy cheap crockery.

The Mamma Nero Diaries will give you a unique understanding of how Anthony developed his strength of character and how it helped him meet the challenges that cancer presented him.

Available in paperback and for Kindle.

COMING SOON

The Italian Cookbook:
It's a Family Thing

Keep an eye on Anthony's website for more details:

www.adhyde.com

ABOUT THE AUTHOR

Anthony Hyde is a second-generation Italian who grew up on the cobbled streets of Manchester... well, when he says on, he really means close by... in a house. He spent most of his childhood watching sci-fi/ fantasy movies and fishing for newts and sticklebacks in the local canal. He dreamt of going to university, meeting and marrying the girl of his dreams, settling down to have a family and living happily ever after... and, of course, becoming an astronaut with magical powers.

One by one his dreams started to come true: he graduated with a degree in physics, met and married the girl of his dreams and had two beautiful girls. Unfortunately, while he was living happily ever after, he was diagnosed with Chronic Myeloid Leukaemia.

This event awakened the writer's voice within him and gave him the inspiration to write *The Leukaemia Diaries*, which is a light-hearted and inspirational account of his experiences from just before being diagnosed with CML through treatment and beyond.

In addition to building his back catalogue with books like *The Mamma Nero Diaries* and *The Italian Cookbook*, he is also working hard on his remaining dreams... especially the one where he develops magical powers.

Website: www.adhyde.com
Facebook: www.facebook.com/ADHydeAuthor
Twitter: twitter.com/adhydeauthor
Instagram: www.instagram.com/adhydeauthor/

Printed in Great Britain
by Amazon

27916502R00066